ANNALS *of* THE NEW YORK ACADEMY OF SCIENCES

VOLUME
1283

ISBN-10: 1-57331-866-3; **ISBN-13:** 978-1-57331-866-2

ISSUE

Translational Immunology in Asia-Oceania

The 5th FIMSA Congress

T0344664

ISSUE EDITOR

Narinder K. Mehra

Annals of the New York Academy of Sciences (ISSN: 0077-8923 [print]; ISSN: 1749-6632 [online]) is published 30 times a year on behalf of the New York Academy of Sciences by Wiley Subscription Services, Inc., a Wiley Company, 111 River Street, Hoboken, NJ 07030-5774.

Mailing: *Annals of the New York Academy of Sciences* is mailed standard rate.

Postmaster: Send all address changes to ANNALS OF THE NEW YORK ACADEMY OF SCIENCES, Journal Customer Services, John Wiley & Sons Inc., 350 Main Street, Malden, MA 02148-5020.

Disclaimer: The publisher, the New York Academy of Sciences, and the editors cannot be held responsible for errors or any consequences arising from the use of information contained in this publication; the views and opinions expressed do not necessarily reflect those of the publisher, the New York Academy of Sciences, and editors, neither does the publication of advertisements constitute any endorsement by the publisher, the New York Academy of Sciences and editors of the products advertised.

Publisher: *Annals of the New York Academy of Sciences* is published by Wiley Periodicals, Inc., Commerce Place, 350 Main Street, Malden, MA 02148; Telephone: 781 388 8200; Fax: 781 388 8210.

Journal Customer Services: For ordering information, claims, and any inquiry concerning your subscription, please go to www.wileycustomerhelp.com/ask or contact your nearest office. *Americas:* Email: cs-journals@wiley.com; Tel:+1 781 388 8598 or 1 800 835 6770 (Toll free in the USA & Canada). *Europe, Middle East, Asia:* Email: cs-journals@wiley. com; Tel: +44 (0) 1865 778315. *Asia Pacific:* Email: cs-journals@wiley.com; Tel: +65 6511 8000. *Japan:* For Japanese speaking support, Email: cs-japan@wiley.com; Tel: +65 6511 8010 or Tel (toll-free): 005 316 50 480. Visit our Online Customer Get-Help available in 6 languages at www.wileycustomerhelp.com.

Information for Subscribers: *Annals of the New York Academy of Sciences* is published in 30 volumes per year. Subscription prices for 2013 are: Print & Online: US$6,053 (US), US$6,589 (Rest of World), €4,269 (Europe), £3,364 (UK). Prices are exclusive of tax. Australian GST, Canadian GST, and European VAT will be applied at the appropriate rates. For more information on current tax rates, please go to www.wileyonlinelibrary.com/tax-vat. The price includes online access to the current and all online back files to January 1, 2009, where available. For other pricing options, including access information and terms and conditions, please visit www.wileyonlinelibrary.com/access.

Delivery Terms and Legal Title: Where the subscription price includes print volumes and delivery is to the recipient's address, delivery terms are Delivered at Place (DAP); the recipient is responsible for paying any import duty or taxes. Title to all volumes transfers FOB our shipping point, freight prepaid. We will endeavour to fulfill claims for missing or damaged copies within six months of publication, within our reasonable discretion and subject to availability.

Back issues: Recent single volumes are available to institutions at the current single volume price from cs-journals@wiley.com. Earlier volumes may be obtained from Periodicals Service Company, 11 Main Street, Germantown, NY 12526, USA. Tel: +1 518 537 4700, Fax: +1 518 537 5899, Email: psc@periodicals.com. For submission instructions, subscription, and all other information visit: www.wileyonlinelibrary.com/journal/nyas.

Production Editors: Kelly McSweeney and Allie Struzik (email: nyas@wiley.com).

Commercial Reprints: Dan Nicholas (email: dnicholas@wiley.com).

Membership information: Members may order copies of *Annals* volumes directly from the Academy by visiting www. nyas.org/annals, emailing customerservice@nyas.org, faxing +1 212 298 3650, or calling 1 800 843 6927 (toll free in the USA), or +1 212 298 8640. For more information on becoming a member of the New York Academy of Sciences, please visit www.nyas.org/membership. Claims and inquiries on member orders should be directed to the Academy at email: membership@nyas.org or Tel: 1 800 843 6927 (toll free in the USA) or +1 212 298 8640.

Printed in the USA by The Sheridan Group.

View *Annals* online at www.wileyonlinelibrary.com/journal/nyas.

Abstracting and Indexing Services: *Annals of the New York Academy of Sciences* is indexed by MEDLINE, Science Citation Index, and SCOPUS. For a complete list of A&I services, please visit the journal homepage at www. wileyonlinelibrary.com/journal/nyas.

Access to *Annals* is available free online within institutions in the developing world through the AGORA initiative with the FAO, the HINARI initiative with the WHO, and the OARE initiative with UNEP. For information, visit www. aginternetwork.org, www.healthinternetwork.org, www.oarescience.org.

Annals of the New York Academy of Sciences accepts articles for Open Access publication. Please visit http://olabout.wiley.com/WileyCDA/Section/id-406241.html for further information about OnlineOpen.

Wiley's Corporate Citizenship initiative seeks to address the environmental, social, economic, and ethical challenges faced in our business and which are important to our diverse stakeholder groups. Since launching the initiative, we have focused on sharing our content with those in need, enhancing community philanthropy, reducing our carbon impact, creating global guidelines and best practices for paper use, establishing a vendor code of ethics, and engaging our colleagues and other stakeholders in our efforts. Follow our progress at www.wiley.com/go/citizenship.

ANNALS OF THE NEW YORK ACADEMY OF SCIENCES

Issue: *Translational Immunology in Asia-Oceania*

A brief history of the Federation of Immunological Societies of Asia-Oceania (FIMSA)

The "5th Congress of the Federation of Immunological Societies of Asia-Oceania" was held on March 14–17, 2012 in New Delhi, India in conjunction with the "39th Annual Conference of the Indian Immunology Society." The theme of the conference was translational immunology in health and disease. The following essay[a] outlines the history of the Federation of Immunological Societies of Asia-Oceania (FIMSA) and its impact on immunological societies throughout Asia-Oceania.

The science of immunology is multidisciplinary and multifaceted, and includes topics that have significant influence in biology and medicine. Although the first Nobel Prize (in Physiology or Medicine) in the field of immunology was given in 1901 to Emil Adolf von Behring for his work on serum therapy, especially in its application against diphtheria, a full understanding of the cellular network and of crosstalk between various immunologically relevant cell types was realized much later. Today, immunology is recognized as a mature scientific discipline that has made remarkable advances in the last 50 years. The fundamental principles of normal immune response are now well understood, and many novel therapies have been developed. Identified areas for growth in the field, however, are in the study of the translational role in human disease. For instance, the underlying pathogenesis of autoimmune and allergic diseases is not fully understood, and, despite the rapid advances in the identification of susceptibility genes for these diseases, the connection between genetics and the pathogenesis of these diseases remains elusive. Vaccine development remains an empirical art, inasmuch as it has proved difficult to apply scientific principles to the development of improved vaccines. As a result, development of effective vaccines against the three most devastating infections, HIV, tuberculosis, and malaria, is still ongoing. Controlling immune responses to newly introduced genes and viral vectors has been a significant problem for gene therapy and is the major reason why all systematic gene therapy protocols have been curtailed. Furthermore, despite the worldwide excitement about the potential of regenerative medicine, stem cell therapies (with the exception of hematopoietic stem cell transplants) will very likely face the daunting problem of rejection; unless we solve this concern, stem cell therapy may never realize its full potential.

The International Union of Immunological Societies (IUIS), the driving force behind improving promotion and understanding of immunology, has worked admirably to achieve its fundamental goal of advancing immunology in many regions of the world. The union already includes more than 50 immunological societies in six continents and has done remarkably well through its committees and various outreach programs. Specifically, it has promoted the establishment of regional federations, which, in turn, have proved useful for maximizing the available resources and promoting career development of young

---

[a]An earlier version of this essay was published online in the FIMSA newsletter 2011/1/26, vol.1: http://message. csmu.edu.tw/ePaper/ePaperBrowse.asp?PublishID=65. This version is published with permission.

doi: 10.1111/nyas.12096

immunologists. Presently, the IUIS has four regional federations under its umbrella, each one committed to the promotion and advancement of immunology in its respective region: the European Federation of Immunological Societies (EFIS), the Latin American Association of Immunology (ALAI), the Federation of African Immunological Societies (FAIS), and the Federation of Immunological Societies of Asia-Oceania (FIMSA). The union held its first international congress in August 1971 in Washington, D.C. Now, four decades later, the union has conducted fourteen such congresses; the 15th and 16th are planned for Milan, Italy in August 2013 and Melbourne, Australia in 2016.

With regard to the Asia-Oceania region, the following statistics are relevant in the context of the promotion of science, in general, and immunology, in particular. Whereas 94% of all scientists in the world live and work in the developed world, only 6% of scientists live and work in the developing countries. Although Asia has nearly two-thirds of the world's population, only a small minority of Asian scientists (with the exception of Japan) are represented in global science meetings. The scientific literature is often full of lead papers from scientists from Europe, North America, Japan, and Australia, with negligible representation from those in Asian countries other than Japan. In the IUIS, while 80–85% of nearly 40,000 IUIS members come from Western countries, only about 15% come from Asian countries, the majority coming from Japan. The situation seems to be changing, however, as was evident by the impressive participation of Asian countries at the last immunology meeting in August 2010 in Kobe, Japan.

An important and noteworthy feature of the Asia-Oceania region is its extraordinary heterogeneity. In addition to the large size of the region, the distances involved are important limiting factors. Scientists in the region have often found it difficult to interact with their counterparts in the West. Thus, for a long time, it was felt that if the national immunology societies of Asia-Oceania region could form a joint forum and function from a common platform, the quantum and progress of the united effort could get augmented, leading to the promotion of immunology using an interdisciplinary approach.

Brief history

The FIMSA was formally established in February 1992 in New Delhi, with the fundamental goals of promoting communication and collaboration among immunologists in the region; organizing training courses, workshops, and other educational programs in all areas of immunology; and supporting exchange among scientists in aid of the advancement of science in the region. The foundation for such a united body had indeed been laid much earlier. In 1990, I became the secretary of the Indian Immunology Society. This was a critical period, inasmuch as the society's bid for holding the 10th International Immunology Congress had to be prepared and, more importantly, presented to the IUIS council for their consideration. I had very little knowledge of IUIS affairs, much less of the role of its regional federations. I later learned that although there were federations established in Europe and Latin America, there was actually none representing immunology societies in Asia-Oceania and the African continent. A chance discussion in our executive meeting convinced us of the need for the establishment of a federation of immunology societies in Asia-Oceania. In fact, we felt that such a federation would be advantageous for the 1998 immunology congress, for which we were seriously preparing a bid document, thanks to the efforts of Professor Pran Talwar, widely regarded as the father of immunology in India.

As secretary of the society, I contacted fellow society heads in countries in the region, informing them of our desire to form a regional federation. By end of 1990, an ad hoc body under the name Asia-Oceania Federation of Immunological Societies (AOFIS) was established, which received active support from all member societies, and the IUIS in particular. Professor Jacob Natvig, then president of the IUIS, played a key role in making this federation a reality (Fig. 1). Jacob invited me to join the IUIS council meeting in Edinburgh, Scotland in September 1990, and to present the concept of the proposed federation; this was further discussed by the council in Helsinki in June 1991. During this period Jacob and I visited a number of countries in the region, meeting society heads and discussing the creation of an Asia-Oceania federation. I was witness to tremendous enthusiasm and sincerity of purpose from Jacob; the excitement naturally passed on to me and, like him, I became passionately involved in the cause. During this process, we received major support from Sir Gustav Nossal (Australia) (Fig. 1) and Professor Tomio Tada (Japan),

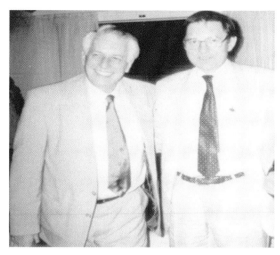

Figure 1. Sir Gustav Nossal (left) and Jacob Natvig (right) provided immense support and encouragement during the founding of the FIMSA.

both of whom were also a great source of inspiration. Sadly enough, we lost Tomio Tada on April 18, 2010 after a brief illness. Tomio was indeed a jewel in the field of immunology, not just for us in the Asia-Oceania region, but the world over.

In February 1992, a planning meeting was convened in New Delhi with the primary objective of formalizing the federation (Fig. 2); it was attended by representatives of six societies that included Roland Scollay (Australia), Wei Feng Chen (Beijing, China), Stitaya Sirisinha (Thailand), Chung-Ming Chang (Taipei, R.O.C.), Tomio Tada (Japan), Indian representatives, and Jacob Natvig (IUIS). Professor G.P. Talwar (India) was asked unanimously to be the first president of the FIMSA; I had the privilege to serve as the founding secretary-general, a position that I held for two terms until January 2000.

Subsequently, the leadership of the FIMSA has been served with distinction by the following presidents: Roland Scollay, Australia (July 1995 to December 1996); Takehiko Sasazuki, Japan (January 1997 to January 2000); Stitiya Sirisinha, Thailand (January 2000 to April 2005); Kiyoshi Takatsu, Japan (April 2005 to October 2008); Nicholas King, Australia (October 2008 to March 2012); and Xuetao Cao, China (March 2012 to the present). The position of the treasurer was occupied first by Chung Ming Chang, Taipei (February 1992 to July 1995), who provided the much-needed initial stability. Subsequently, Chia Li Yu, Taipei (July 1995 to June 1998), Masayuki Miyasaka, Japan (June 1998 to December 1999, and January 2000 to October 2008), and Shigeo Koyasu, Japan (October 2008 to the present) have served with distinction. Following my tenure as secretary-general, several eminent persons filled that position: Lindsay Dent, Australia (January 2000 to April 2005), Sansanee Chaiyaroj, Thailand (April 2005 to October 2008), and Gregory Tsay, Taipei (October 2008 to the present). In addition, Wei Feng Chen (Beijing, China), Stitaya Sirisinha (Thailand), Tai You Ha (Korea), Narinder Mehra (India), Sansanee Chaiyaroj (Thailand), and Xuetao Cao (China) have served as vice presidents.

At present, the FIMSA comprises 12 societies, each recognized by, and affiliated with, the IUIS. These include the Australasian Society for Immunology; the Chinese Society for Immunology; the Indian Immunology Society; the Japanese Society for Immunology; the Korean Association of Immunologists; the Society for Immunology located in Taipei; the Allergy, Asthma, and Immunology Society of Thailand; the Hong Kong Society for Immunology; the Iranian Society of Immunology, the Singaporean Society for Immunology; the Allergy and Immunology Society of Sri Lankan; and the Papua, New Guinea Immunology Association. In addition, the immunology societies in Bangladesh, the Commonwealth of Independent States, and Russia have observer status, pending their fulfillment of IUIS criteria to become full members. Some societies, like those in Russia and Israel, are observers of the FIMSA because of their geographic

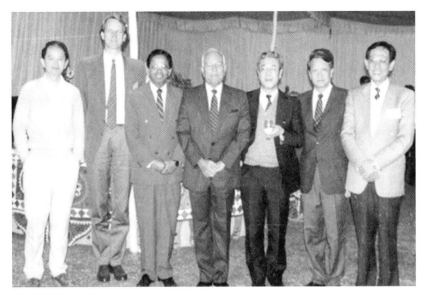

Figure 2. Participants at the planning meeting during the establishment of the FIMSA in New Delhi, February 1992. Left to right: Wei Feng Chen (China), Roland Scollay (Australia), Narinder Mehra (India), Pran Talwar (India), Tomio Tada (Japan), Stitaya Sirisinha (Thailand), and Chung Ming Chang (Taiwan, R.O.C).

location in Asia. We hope that in due course, immunology societies or research groups will be established in several other countries in the region. It is our hope that this network will increase the understanding of biomedical issues in Asia and continue to encourage further research in biotechnology and immunology.

Objectives and purpose

The FIMSA was formed to foster the development of immunology in the region. To this end, the federation promotes close contact and interaction among immunological societies in the Asia-Oceania region and facilitates the exchange of scientific information and personnel. The FIMSA is a nonprofit organization, and its activities are consistent with the guidelines of the IUIS. Its specific objectives are to (1) promote communication and collaboration among immunologists in the region; (2) organize workshops and conferences in the field of immunology; (3) conduct educational programs and training courses; (4) facilitate the exchange of technologies within the region; and (5) support the publication of journals and monographs.

FIMSA congresses

The FIMSA has taken steps to initiate interaction among immunologists in the region by promoting basic and advanced training courses for postdoctoral and midcareer scientists and by organizing international congresses at regular intervals. The historic inaugural FIMSA congress was successfully held in December 1996 in Adelaide, Australia, with Lindsay Dent as the organizing chair (Fig. 3). The second FIMSA congress was organized by Stitaya Sirisinha and his team of dedicated workers in Bangkok, Thailand on January 23–27, 2000. Professor Wei Feng Chen was the driving force behind the third congress held in Hangzhou, China in April 2005, while the fourth congress was held in Taipei, (October 17–21, 2008) under the leadership of Gregory Tsay and his colleagues. The fifth congress was held in New Delhi on March 14–17, 2012 (www.fimsa2012.com); Narinder Mehra was president.

Since the FIMSA came into existence the region has hosted two IUIS International Congresses of Immunology—the 10th congress in New Delhi, India (November 1–6, 1998) and the 14th congress in Kobe, Japan (August 22–27, 2010). The region will host the 16th congress in the vibrant city of Melbourne

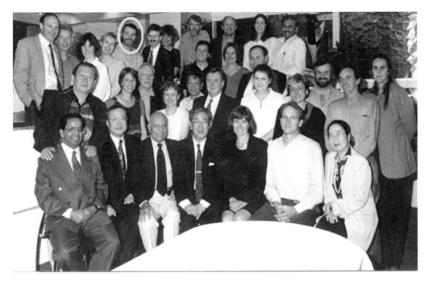

Figure 3. Group photograph of FIMSA officers and congress organizers taken during the "1st FIMSA Congress of Immunology" in Adelaide, Australia, December 1996. Dr. Lindsay Dent who organized the congress and then became secretary-general of the federation is seen (circled) in the top row.

in 2016. Thus, the FIMSA is well on its way toward achieving its goal of contributing actively to the growth of immunology in the Asia-Oceania region.

Training courses

One of the major activities of the FIMSA has been the provision of educational opportunities to young immunologists and the fostering of international cooperation in the region through major advanced training courses. These courses are meant to integrate high-level science, technical advancement, and a basic understanding of immunology. The course participants come from a broad range of backgrounds, and each course has a specific focus that depends on regional needs and requirements.

The FIMSA has already conducted eleven such formal training courses throughout the region: (1) Brisbane, Australia, October 9–15, 1994 (course convener: Professor Ian Frazer), which had almost 40 participants, five of whom were sponsored by the FIMSA and the IUIS; (2) Beijing, China, October 21–27, 1996 (course convener: Wei Feng Chen), which had a total of 133 participants, 10 of whom were sponsored by FIMSA; (3) Hong Kong, June 21–26, 1998 (course conveners: Davina Opstelten and Pak Leong Lim), with 115 participants, including 32 from 10 countries outside Hong Kong; (4) New Delhi, India, March 5–9, 2001 (course convener: Narinder Mehra), with 102 participants from 12 countries; (5) Taipei, Taiwan, R.O.C, September 23–28, 2001 (course convener: Gregory Tsay), with more than 100 participants, including those from mainland China, Hong Kong, and several other Asian countries; (6) Ayutthya, Thailand, October 20–25, 2002 (course chairs: Stitaya Sirisinha and Sansanee Chaiyaroj), with 175 delegates from 32 institutes; (7) Adelaide, Australia, December 7–10, 2004 (course director: Lindsay Dent), with 107 delegates from 12 countries; (8) New Delhi, India, March 1–5, 2006 (course director: Narinder Mehra), with 121 delegates from 13 countries; (9) Jeju Island, Korea, February 1–4, 2007 (organized by the Korean Association of Immunologists); (10) Tangalooma Island, Australia, December 3–6, 2009 (course director: Simon Apte); and (11) New Delhi, India, March 18–20, 2012 (course chairs: Narinder Mehra and Gurvinder Kaur). Through these educational courses, the FIMSA has been successful in achieving its basic objective of providing an interactive platform for young researchers from varying cultural backgrounds.

Over the years, the FIMSA courses have been extremely popular, as seen from the large number of applications received; organizers have often had to accommodate many more students than originally planned for. The course faculty has always been carefully selected to provide the broadest possible perspective. To this end, the European Federation of Immunological Societies has shown their cooperation by providing speaker support, as has the Japanese Society for Immunology and the Australasian Society for Immunology.

Acknowledgments

I wish to thank a large number of colleagues and eminent immunologists in the region for their selfless service to the FIMSA. Space constraints do not permit me to name all of them individually, but their contributions have been enormous and praiseworthy. I give my utmost regards to Jacob Natvig, who provided the initial momentum for the founding of the FIMSA, and to the three stalwart immunologists of the region, Tomio Tada (Japan), Gustav Nossal (Australia), and Pran Talwar (India) for their advice. I also gratefully acknowledge the support and encouragement provided by the Indian Immunology Society.

Narinder K. Mehra
Department of Transplant Immunology and Immunogenetics
All India Institute of Medical Sciences, New Delhi, India

Ann. N.Y. Acad. Sci. ISSN 0077-8923

Immunology and world health: key contributions from the global community

G. J. V. Nossal

Department of Pathology, The University of Melbourne, Melbourne, Australia

Address for correspondence: Sir Gustav Nossal, Department of Pathology, The University of Melbourne, Vic. 3010, Australia. gnossal@bigpond.net.au

The contributions of immunology to world health must be seen in the context of the severe disadvantage prevailing in many countries. Low life expectancy, high infant and maternal mortality rates, and continued prevalence of infections as causes of preventable deaths highlight what vaccines can do to improve the situation. This paper will briefly review some major new international health programs, including the GAVI Alliance; the Global Polio Eradication Initiative; the Global Fund to Fight AIDS, Tuberculosis and Malaria; the President's Emergency Plan for AIDS Relief; and the Global Malaria Action Plan. It will also outline the state of research progress for vaccines that are not yet licensed but that, in many cases, appear within reach. Of course, vaccines are not the be-all and the end-all of global health, so brief reference will be made to nutrition, vector biology and control, and the emergence of noncommunicable diseases as threats.

Keywords: foreign aid; vaccines; poliomyelitis; HIV; AIDS; malaria

Introduction

A new breeze is blowing in international health as both philanthropists and governments realize how much can be done to alleviate the grievous health problems in the poorest countries.[1] To understand the contribution that immunology can make, we must first realize the scale of the problem, then recall that infections still dominate in causing premature deaths, and then ponder what steps can be taken both to bring newer vaccines to developing countries and to sponsor research into vaccines primarily of value to the poor. This brief essay seeks to embed immunological research and development within the wider universe of social justice and economic development.

Mortality statistics highlight huge global inequities

The most dramatic single statistic highlighting the inequities between rich and poor countries is life expectancy. In the industrialized countries, this has risen remarkably over the last 50 years. Pooling statistics for men and women, life expectancy at birth in Sweden has risen from 73 in 1960 to 81 in 2011; in Australia, from 71 to 82; in the United States from 71 to 78; and in Japan from 68 to 81. This approximately 10-year extension has not been granted to the developing countries. The worst statistics come from sub-Saharan African. Life expectancy at birth has gone from 45 to 39 in Zambia and from 33 to 38 in Angola. In 2011, the lowest national life expectancy was only 46% of the highest.

The number of deaths under the age of five years per thousand live births is often used as a surrogate of the efficacy of health systems. Table 1 compares rates in 1960 versus 2009 in eight countries. Overall, the improvement has been remarkable. The countries that have only recently become industrialized lead the way, such as India, which has shown an almost fivefold improvement. Once again, the sub-Saharan African countries lag behind.

Over the last decade, worldwide improvement in mortality has occurred at the rate of 2.8% per year. At the same time, the worst national mortality remains 78-fold higher than the best. Pneumonia accounts for 1.5 million deaths per year, diarrheal

doi: 10.1111/nyas.12035

Table 1. Deaths under five years per 1,000 live births

	1960	2009
Singapore	28.6	2.3
Japan	25.8	2.8
Australia	19.8	4.7
USA	25.4	6.3
Angola	199.9	180.2
Zambia	126.6	101.2
India	140.1	30.1
Nigeria	164.0	94.3

NOTES: 2009 mortality worst to best: 78-fold difference. Last decade world improvement: 2.8% per annum. Pneumonia 1.5 million; diarrhea 740,000; malaria 670,000 deaths.

diseases for 740,000, and malaria for 670,000. Two-thirds of these deaths are preventable.

A third stunning statistic, not directly linked to immunology, concerns deaths in pregnancy and childbirth. Such maternal mortality has become vanishingly rare in the richer countries. In fact, when such deaths occur, they are usually related to some underlying disease of the mother that has nothing to do with the pregnancy. In 2008, Italy exhibited the lowest maternal mortality, with 3.9 deaths per 100,000 live births, while Afghanistan had the highest, with 1,575. This appalling 404-fold difference illustrates the difficulty of coping with hemorrhage, sepsis, or obstructed labor in remote, resource-poor regions. In the last 20 years, global maternal mortality has improved at only 1.4% per year.

The role of aid in improving health

While national efforts are absolutely essential, there is no doubt that international aid has played a significant role in improving health.[2] Figure 1 tells an interesting story. In 1960, there were 20 million deaths in children under five but in 2010 only about eight million. The figure, taken from statistics from the Bill & Melinda Gates Foundation, projects two scenarios out to 2025: continued improvement along the same lines or no change. Aggregating all the deaths in the triangular area between the two projections, we reach the conclusion that scaling up basic health interventions could prevent 27 million child deaths by 2025. Such a result would likely require vaccine development, malaria prevention and

treatment, better treatment of pneumonia and diarrhea, and better practices in newborn care.

A stated goal of the United Nations, at the prompting of former Prime Minister of Canada Lester Pearson, is that all industrialized countries devote 0.7% of their gross national income (GNI) to official development assistance (ODA). In 2010 the global total of ODA was U.S. $128.5 billion, or just 0.32% of the relevant countries' GNI. Only five countries reached or exceeded the benchmark: Denmark, Norway, Sweden, the Netherlands, and Luxembourg. My own country, Australia, currently devotes 0.35% of its GNI to ODA, though it has pledged to go to 0.5% by 2016/17. The health component of ODA varies from country to country, generally representing 7–15% of the total. Over the past decade or so, large programs have finally emerged with annual budgets measured in the billions rather than the millions. These include the GAVI Alliance; the Global Polio Eradication Initiative; the Global Fund to Fight AIDS, Tuberculosis and Malaria; the President's Emergency Plan for AIDS Relief; and the Global Malaria Action Plan.

The GAVI alliance

The GAVI Alliance, formerly known as the Global Alliance for Vaccines and Immunization, was launched at the World Economic Forum in Davos, Switzerland, in January 2000. It seeks to bring vaccines to the 72 poorest countries in the world, initially targeting those with a GDP per capita of less than $1,000 per year, later raised to $1,500 per year.[3] The chief goals of the GAVI Alliance are increasing infant coverage with the six common childhood vaccines (diphtheria, pertussis, tetanus, poliomyelitis, measles, BCG); supporting the introduction of newer vaccines; improving safe injection practices and syringe and needle disposal; and promoting research and development of new or improved vaccines. The GAVI Alliance was initially supported by a grant of $750,000,000 from the Bill & Melinda Gates Foundation but now also receives extensive support from many aid agencies, other foundations, and funds, and the annual budget exceeds $1 billion and continues to rise. Through the end of 2011, 326 million additional children have been immunized, an estimated 5.5 million deaths have been averted, and infant coverage with the basic vaccines has risen from 66% to 82% in GAVI-eligible countries.

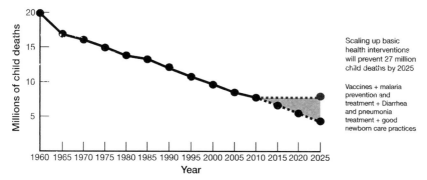

Figure 1. Aid has helped reduce child deaths dramatically, and can continue to do so. Source: Johns Hopkins Bloomberg School of Public Health; Bill & Melinda Gates Foundation estimates.

The introduction of newer vaccines is best understood in a historic context. The first major push was for the inclusion of hepatitis B, largely to expand a preexisting World Health Organization (WHO) program. Hepatitis B is not a major killer of children but it causes chronic infection that can lead to liver cirrhosis and primary hepatocellular carcinoma. The second new GAVI vaccine was against *Haemophilus influenzae* type b, a cause of pneumonia and meningitis, included because a new carbohydrate–protein conjugate vaccine had proven so successful in industrialized countries.[4] The third vaccine, against yellow fever, was a very good but underused older vaccine. It is relevant in only some countries.

From there, the range of new vaccines expanded rapidly though it has not been feasible to roll out every vaccine in every country because of cost pressures. Probably the most important is the multivalent conjugate vaccine for *Streptococcus pneumoniae*. Special financing methods are in place to bring pneumococcal vaccines on board as rapidly as possible and to persuade pharmaceutical companies to lower their prices.[5] In the longer term, vaccines composed of highly conserved pneumococcal proteins, capable of covering all serotypes, will be required. The most important viral cause of diarrhea is rotavirus. Two first world rotavirus vaccines are being deployed and a cheaper Indian vaccine is on the threshold. Though these vaccines are not as successful in a developing country setting as in the West,[6] they are nevertheless powerful public health tools against this serious killer. GAVI also has early plans to include human papilloma virus vaccines to fight cervical cancer and *Rubella* vaccine to prevent birth defects caused by the virus in early pregnancy.

GAVI's work in injection safety rotates around the use of "uniject" and "autodisable" injection equipment and the promotion of efficient disposal of syringes and needles,[6] all of which aim to prevent illicit use in the drug trade. There is also work underway to safeguard the cold chain and to train leaders of immunization programs. Research and development has now largely been delegated to a series of independent product development partnerships, each still retaining significant Gates Foundation funding and influence. One successful example has been the African Meningitis Vaccine Programme.[7] This is a joint venture between WHO and the Seattle-based nongovernmental organization PATH. It aims to prevent the horrible recurrent epidemics of meningococcal meningitis across the so-called meningitis belt of sub-Saharan Africa. This runs from Senegal in the west to Ethiopia in the east and comprises 25 countries with a combined population of 300 million. These epidemics are chiefly of *Neisseria meningitidis* serogroup A. The disease has a case fatality rate of 10–20% with many more subjects suffering serious sequelae including mental retardation. It is so feared by the population that health services are virtually paralyzed because outbreak control dominates all other efforts. The worst affected countries are Burkina Faso, Chad, Ethiopia, and Niger. An open competition was engendered whereby vaccine companies in industrialized and developing countries were offered a seeding grant of $70 million by the Gates Foundation and asked for their best price to produce a carbohydrate–protein conjugate vaccine for meningococcus A. The Serum Institute of India in Pune won the competition with a bid of 50 cents per dose of vaccine. After a great deal of collaboration and technology transfer, they came up with a licensed vaccine in 2009 and a projected vaccine price of 40 cents per dose. This was progressively rolled out in Burkina Faso, Mali, Niger, Chad, Cameroon, and northern Nigeria. Antibody responses were much better than those to the older carbohydrate vaccine. In Burkina Faso, where most of the population was covered, there were only four cases of meningitis in 2011, and all of these were in unimmunized people. The vaccine has reached 55 million people so far and should reach most of the 300 million by 2016.

Global poliomyelitis eradication initiative

Following the successful eradication of smallpox, certified in 1980,[8] it seemed logical to target another vaccine-preventable disease for global eradication, and poliomyelitis was chosen. The initiative, a partnership among Rotary International, WHO, UNICEF, and a number of other organizations, was launched in 1988.[9] A number of key strategies were established relatively early. The Sabin oral poliomyelitis vaccine was chosen rather than the Salk injectable vaccine for a number of reasons, including the lower cost and the greater ease of administration, particularly important since many Rotarian volunteers were to be used in the program. High routine infant coverage with the six common vaccines was encouraged but it was determined that not all children would be reached. Therefore a new stratagem was the creation of national immunization days (NID). Amid considerable media publicity, great involvement of civil society, and patronage by the head of state, first lady, or other high dignitary, a particular day was identified as an NID for a given country, and all children under the age of five, regardless of previous immunization history, were encouraged to line up and get their polio drops. Frequently, vitamin A was also administered, at the low price of two cents per dose. Often, a second NID was called for two weeks later, resulting in high population coverage.

Effective surveillance for the detection of polio cases became particularly important, especially when only a small number occurred. Each new case

of acute flaccid paralysis had to provide two stool samples that were sent to accredited laboratories for the isolation of the polio virus. In fact, the low number of nonpolio cases of paralysis can be taken as a measure of the excellence of surveillance, because the incidence appears to vary relatively little. A further important step is the prompt control of any small outbreak of polio that may occur after apparent eradication. This is achieved by the widespread use of two doses of vaccine two weeks apart around the index case.

These strategies have been very successful. The incidence of polio cases has been reduced by over 99%. In 2010, there were 874 confirmed cases globally and in 2011 only 650. India's unswerving commitment and strong leadership resulted in no new cases seen since January 13, 2011—this populous country is now polio free. There are only three countries in which polio has never been eradicated: Pakistan, Afghanistan, and Nigeria. Unfortunately, in three countries polio transmission has been reestablished after prior eradication and case importation: Chad, the Democratic Republic of Congo, and Angola. Finally, there are small importation-caused outbreaks, which have been rapidly controlled in most cases. There is still some distance to travel before the final goal is reached.

The price of failure in eradication would indeed be high. Apart from the loss of prestige, the financial implications are dire. The world is currently spending $1 billion per year on the program for a minute public health gain. Of the $9.5 billion total cost since 1988, Rotary International has contributed over $1 billion and the Gates Foundation $400 million. The Strategic Advisory Group of Experts guiding WHO on immunization has stated that failure to eradicate polio would constitute the most expensive public health failure in history, and the independent Global Polio Eradication Monitoring Board declared in February 2012 that the present situation should be treated as a major emergency, a position confirmed by the World Health Assembly. Margaret Chan, director-general of the WHO, cites polio eradication as her top operational priority. The economic benefits of eradication have been estimated at $40 to $50 billion.

The global response to the AIDS pandemic

The world's response to the AIDS pandemic has been to launch two multibillion dollar programs:

the Global Fund to Fight AIDS, Tuberculosis and Malaria, and the President's Emergency Fund for AIDS Relief. Together, these are budgeted at around $12 billion per year, dwarfing all other health programs. As a result, 6.5 million people in low and middle income countries are receiving highly active antiretroviral therapy, transforming their lives. There are at least 600,000 cases per year of treatments to prevent mother to child transmission of the virus, a highly effective and low cost health initiative. There is now good evidence that the pandemic has peaked, with fewer new cases per year. Apart from helping the patient, treatment of AIDS cases lowers the viral burden and thus the likelihood of transmission from that person. There is still some distance to go, however, before everyone needing therapy receives it.

The Global Malaria Action Plan and global Stop TB Partnership

The Global Malaria Action Plan seeks to deliver effective prevention and treatment and is implemented by the Roll Back Malaria partnership. The ambitious plan is to reduce malaria cases to 25% of year 2000 levels by 2015, to eliminate malaria in 8–10 countries by that date, and to have "near zero" deaths by 2015. The primary tools for prevention are insecticide-impregnated bednets, which have been highly effective (at least 240 million have been distributed so far); indoor residual insecticide spraying; and intermittent preventive treatment with artemisinine combination therapy for children and pregnant women in high transmission settings. Better case management of actual cases is also envisaged. The plan is receiving about $2 billion annually at the moment and ambitious fund-raising targets have been set for 2012–2015.

The global Stop TB Partnership, which includes over 1,200 organizations, seeks to unite all the efforts to fight tuberculosis. While directly observed treatment short-course (DOTS) remains central, the plan also foresees significant advances in research and development focused on new diagnostics, new drugs, and new vaccines. High priority will be given to the twin dilemmas of drug-resistant TB and the combination of TB and HIV. From 1995 to 2009, 49 million TB patients were treated with DOTS, 41 million of them successfully. It is hoped that a therapy will eventually be developed that takes only two weeks.

Progress toward vaccines for HIV/AIDS, malaria, and tuberculosis

The field of vaccines for HIV/AIDS was at last given some encouragement when the RV 144 phase III trial of Sanofi Pasteur's prime-boost vaccine, which involves priming with the ALVAC vector and boosting with the AIDSVAX gp 120 protein, gave modest protection.[10] Sixteen thousand Thai volunteers were involved, and the vaccine provided protection for 31.2% from HIV infection (51 infections versus 74 in placebo controls, $P = 0.04$). However, no lowering of the virus set point was noted in the vaccine group. Analysis of the results suggested that relatively high levels of antibody against the V1/V2 region of the Env protein may have been a factor in protection.[11]

As of May 2012, no other phase III trials are in place. The most advanced trial is a phase IIb safety and efficacy trial (HVTN 505) of a vaccine involving three priming injections of DNA over an eight-week period followed by a single boost of an adenovirus 5-vectored vaccine. This trial began in June 2009 and will involve 2,200 men aged 18–50, all of whom are circumcised and seronegative for antibodies to Ad 5. The men are from 18 U.S. cities; results are expected in 2013. There are two other ongoing phase II studies and a further one expected to start in September 2012. There are 41 phase I studies, most of them prime-boost, ongoing in various parts of the world. Furthermore, at least four neutralizing human-monoclonal antibodies are in preclinical studies for passive immunization.

The furthest advanced malaria-vaccine candidate is RTS,S from GlaxoSmithKline.[12] The phase III clinical trial involves 15,460 children and 11 centers in seven African countries. The vaccine targets the circumsporozoite antigen of *Plasmodium falciparum* and uses the AS01 adjuvant. This involves four different principles of adjuvanticity: hepatitis B-like polymeric particles are constructed; liposomes are used; monophosphoryl lipid A is included; and the saponin QS 21 is added. The first results, published in October 2011, showed that three doses of RTS,S in 5- to 17-month-old children reduced clinical malaria and severe malaria by 56% and 47%, respectively, over a 12-month period. Results in 6- to 12-week-old infants are expected by the end of 2012.

The World Health Organization's malaria vaccine rainbow table summarizes all ongoing malaria vaccine trials, grouped under the headings preerythrocytic, blood stage, sexual stage, and *P. vivax* projects. Furthermore, an excellent review based on the table has recently appeared.[13] It documents how over 40 malaria vaccine candidates have reached the clinical trial stage.

Tuberculosis vaccine research has also been very active.[14] There are five candidates in phase II clinical trials. AERAS-402/Crucell Ad 35 uses a replication-deficient adenovirus against which there is little pre-existent antibody as a vector and coding for the TB antigens 85A, 85B, and TB 10.4. This formulation induces a high CD8+ T cell response in individuals previously immunized with BCG. Three trial sites in Kenya, South Africa, and Mozambique are involved; results will be known in 2014. AERAS-485/MVA 85A uses modified vaccinia Ankara as a vector for 85A, and some 2,750 South African infants previously immunized with BCG are involved in the trial. This formulation induces high levels of polyfunctional CD4+ T cells. It is also being evaluated in HIV-seropositive adults. Results are expected between 2012 and 2014.

GlaxoSmithKline is evaluating GSKM72 in clinical trials. This is a subunit vaccine that uses a recombinant fusion protein of antigens tb32 and tb39 formulated in AS02a adjuvant. Strong cellular and humoral immunity is induced.

VPM 1002 has recently entered a phase II trial involving 48 infants in South Africa. Pioneered by Stefan Kaufmann in Germany, it is a genetically modified *Mycobacterium bovis* and is intended to replace the present BCG.

The State Serum Institute in Denmark and the pharmaceutical firm Intercell are promoting the H1IC vaccine to phase II trial in HIV-seropositive individuals. This subunit vaccine consists of antigens 85B and ESAT-6 and the adjuvant IC 31. Further trials are planned in healthy adolescents. The studies are in South Africa and Tanzania and first results will be available in 2013.

Some further vaccine challenges

Table 2 presents some of the challenges for vaccinology in the immediate future.[1,15] Some, such as the Vi-protein conjugate for *S. typhi*, are already realities in developing countries, though not yet licensed for global use. Some appear quite close, such as the

Table 2. Some further vaccine challenges

Bacterial	Protein for *meningococcus* B
	Protein for *pneumococcus*
	Various approaches for group A *streptococcus*
	Vi-conjugate for *Salmonella typhi*
	Live attenuated or subunit vaccines for *Shigella*
	Live attenuated or subunit vaccines for *Helicobacter pylori*
Viral	Dengue (Sanofi Pasteur phase III end 2012)
	Cheaper rotavirus–India prominent (Bharat, Shanta, Serum Institute of India)
	Broadly active influenza
	Inhalable measles
Parasitic	More complete malaria vaccine (liver, blood, sexual stage antigens)
	Protozoa: leishmaniasis, trypanosomiasis
	Metazoa: schistosomiasis, hookworm, Onchocerciasis, *Taenia*

Novartis *meningococcus* B vaccine, yet many remain some distance away. A further conundrum will be how to pay for so many vaccines. New modes of delivery may well be required, as mothers may be reluctant to expose their infants to still more needle pricks. That being said, the future for global vaccinology research and development is truly exciting.

The Gates Foundation is not limiting its efforts to immunization. It has a program actively researching genetically modified staple crops of enhanced nutritional value, with higher levels of key vitamins and minerals and higher content of proteins rich in essential amino acids. It invests in vector biology and control. One exciting program, run by Scott O'Neill and Ary Hoffmann, seeks to fight dengue.[16] *Aedes aegypti* mosquitoes are infected with *Wolbachia* bacteria harmless to humans; as this infection spreads in the mosquito population, it shortens the mosquito life span just enough so that the dengue virus cannot mature. Thus, spread of dengue is impeded.

As countries progress down the development pathway, more people adopt sedentary lifestyles and, in some cases, Western diets. So diseases like cardiovascular disease, obesity, and diabetes become manifest. For the emerging middle class in China and India, for example, these diseases have become more significant than infections. Public health programs should note this shift. Finally, mental health problems often go unnoticed in developing countries;

for example, unipolar depression is a particularly common and vexing problem.

For the next 20 years at least, the lure of new and improved vaccines will be one of the central preoccupations in public health. This overview has only scratched the surface. There are challenges aplenty.

Conflicts of interest

The author declares no conflicts of interest.

References

1. Nossal, G.J.V. 2011. Vaccines and future global health needs. *Phil. Trans. R. Soc. B.* **366:** 2833–2840.
2. Moxon, E.R., P. Das, B. Greenwood, *et al.* 2011. A call to action for the new decade of vaccines. *Lancet* **378:** 298–302.
3. Lob-Levyt, J. 2011. Contribution of the GAVI Alliance to improving health and reducing poverty. *Phil. Trans. R. Soc. B.* **366:** 2743–2747.
4. Heath, P.T. 1998. *Haemophilus influenzae* type b conjugate vaccines: a review of efficacy data. *Pediatr. Infect. Dis. J.* **17**(Suppl)**:** S117–122.
5. Birn, A.-E. & J. Lexchin. 2011. The GAVI Alliance, AMCs and improving immunization coverage through public sector vaccine production in the global south. *Hum. Vacc.* **7:** 291–292.
6. Armah, G.E., R.F. Breiman, M.D. Tapia, *et al.* 2012. Immunogenicity of the pentavalent rotavirus vaccine in African infants. *Vaccine* **30**(Suppl 1)**:** A86–A93.
7. LaForce, F.M., N. Ravenscroft, M. Djingarey & S. Vivivani. 2009. Epidemic meningitis due to group A *Neisseria meningitidis* in the African meningitis belt: a persistent problem with an imminent solution. *Vaccine* **27**(Suppl 2)**:** B13–B19.
8. Fenner, F. 1982. A successful eradication campaign. Global eradication of smallpox. *Rev. Infect. Dis.* **4:** 916–930.
9. Global Polio Eradication Initiative. Report by the WHO Secretariat to the 60th World Health Assembly. Poliomyelitis: mechanism for management of potential risks to eradication. http://www.polioeradication.org/content/general/WHA61_Resolution_English.pdf (accessed Dec 15, 2011).
10. Rerks-Ngarm, S., P. Pitisuttithum, S. Nitayaphan, *et al.* 2009. Vaccination with ALVAC and AIDSVAX to prevent HIV-1 infection in Thailand. *N. Engl. J. Med.* **361:** 2209–2220.
11. Haynes, B.F., P.B. Gilbert, M.J. McElrath, et al. 2012. Immune-correlates analysis of an HIV-1 vaccine efficacy trial. *N. Engl. J. Med.* **366:** 1275–1286.
12. Bejon, P., J. Lusingu, A. Olotu, *et al.* 2008. Efficacy of RTS,S/AS01E vaccine against malaria in children 5 to 17 months of age. *N. Engl. J. Med.* **359:** 2521–2532.
13. Schwartz, L., G.V. Brown, B. Genton & V.S. Moorthy. 2012. A review of malaria vaccine clinical projects based on the WHO Rainbow Table. *Malaria J.* **11:** 11.
14. McShane, H. 2011. Tuberculosis vaccines: beyond bacille Calmette–Guérin. *Phil. Trans. R. Soc. B.* **366:** 2782–2789.
15. Rappuoli, R., S. Black & P.H. Lambert. 2011. Vaccine discovery and translation of new vaccine technology. *Lancet* **378:** 360–368.
16. Hoffmann, A.A., B.L. Montgomery, J. Popovici, *et al.* 2011. Successful establishment of *Wolbachia* in *Aedes* populations to suppress dengue transmission. *Nature* **476:** 454–457.

Ann. N.Y. Acad. Sci. ISSN 0077-8923

ANNALS OF THE NEW YORK ACADEMY OF SCIENCES
Issue: *Translational Immunology in Asia-Oceania*

The life of regulatory T cells

Iris K. Gratz,[1] Michael D. Rosenblum,[1] and Abul K. Abbas[2]

[1]Department of Dermatology, [2]Department of Pathology, University of California San Francisco—School of Medicine, San Francisco, California

Address for correspondence: Abul K. Abbas, M.B.B.S., Department of Pathology, University of California San Francisco, 505 Parnassus Avenue, Suite M590, San Francisco, CA 94143-0511. abul.abbas@ucsf.edu

Foxp3$^+$ regulatory T (T$_{reg}$) cells are essential for maintaining self-tolerance and preventing autoimmune reactions. T$_{reg}$ cells arise as a consequence of self-antigen recognition during the maturation of cells in the thymus, and also following self-antigen recognition in the periphery. Both thymic and peripherally generated T$_{reg}$ cells respond to antigen recognition by expanding in number, increasing their suppressive activity, and accumulating in the tissue where the antigen is located. A fraction of these activated "effector" T$_{reg}$ cells survive even in the absence of antigen expression and continue to control inflammatory reaction in the tissues, thus functioning as a population of "memory" T$_{reg}$ cells. Antigen exposure and the presence of IL-2 are key determinants in the generation of memory T$_{reg}$ cells. These results provide a foundation for studying the role of memory T$_{reg}$ cells in controlling and treating autoimmune disorders and for testing the hypothesis that defects in the generation and maintenance of these cells underlie chronic, relapsing inflammatory diseases.

Keywords: regulatory T cells; memory cells; tolerance; regulation

Introduction

Although many diverse regulatory lymphocyte populations have been described, the one whose essential role is best established is the Foxp3$^+$ regulatory T (T$_{reg}$) cell population. This conclusion is based largely on the severe autoimmune phenotypes of humans and mice with mutations or targeted deletions of the *Foxp3* gene. It is now known that there are two principal pathways for the generation of these T$_{reg}$ cells. The majority arise during T cell maturation in the thymus, where high-avidity recognition of self-antigen leads to the development of Foxp3$^+$ T$_{reg}$ cells. The mechanisms that determine the choice between generation of these T$_{reg}$ cells and deletion (negative selection) of self-reactive T cells are still not defined. These thymus-derived T$_{reg}$ cells (here referred to as tT$_{reg}$ cells) have also been called "natural" T$_{reg}$ cells. The second pathway of T$_{reg}$ cell generation is in the periphery, when mature, naive CD4 T cells encounter persistent self-antigens. Some of these T cells do not become anergic or die but instead are converted into long-lived T$_{reg}$ cells. These peripherally derived T$_{reg}$ cells (here referred to as pT$_{reg}$ cells) have also been called "adaptive."[1] With the exception of colonic T$_{reg}$ cells, of which many are pT$_{reg}$ cells,[2] it has been suggested that the majority of Foxp3$^+$ T$_{reg}$ cells are thymus derived. However, this has proven difficult to establish with confidence because of the lack of definitive markers for pT$_{reg}$ cells. Although some of the biochemical and functional differences between thymic and peripheral T$_{reg}$ cells have been established, it becomes more and more clear that the suppressive function and the overall expression profile are largely similar.[3,4] Even though some of the requirements for TCR signaling events are similar for tT$_{reg}$ and pT$_{reg}$ cells (e.g., active NF-κB pathway and low AKT/metabolic activation and low ERK/MAPK activity), the precise conditions required for peripheral generation of pT$_{reg}$ cells *in vivo* are still largely undefined.[5–9] Some of the important knowns and unknowns of T$_{reg}$ cell differentiation, stability, and function have been reviewed recently.[10,11]

Responses of T$_{reg}$ cells to a self-antigen

In order to explore the responses of different T cell populations to a tissue self-antigen, we have developed an experimental model in which a known protein, ovalbumin (Ova), is expressed as a tetracycline-inducible antigen in the epidermis.[12]

doi: 10.1111/nyas.12011

In these mice, the antigen is also constitutively expressed in the thymus and induces a large population of Foxp3$^+$ T$_{reg}$ cells when the antigen-expressing mice are crossed with mice expressing a transgenic T cell receptor (TCR) specific for Ova. In addition, by crossing the antigen-expressing mice with TCRα$^{-/-}$ mice to prohibit the development of antigen-specific tT$_{reg}$ cells we obtained a well-defined system in which we can study pT$_{reg}$ cell development from Foxp3$^-$ donor T cells. In summary, our system has allowed us to study responses of both thymic and peripheral T$_{reg}$ cells to tissue self-antigen, and extend earlier studies based on a model of systemic Ova expression.

Thymic T$_{reg}$ cells

Induction of cutaneous Ova in antigen × TCR transgenic mice results in a severe but self-limiting inflammatory skin disease.[12] Two aspects of this disease raise interesting questions. First, the disease develops despite the presence of abundant Ova-specific T$_{reg}$ cells (as many as 40% of the antigen-specific T cells). Second, the disease resolves spontaneously despite continuous antigen expression, and resolution is dependent on CD25$^+$ Foxp3$^+$ T$_{reg}$ cells. These results raise two key questions, Why do T$_{reg}$ cells fail to prevent disease onset, and How do they acquire the ability to "cure" the disease? The answer turns out to be that before peripheral antigen expression Foxp3$^+$ cells are not highly suppressive. After encountering their cognate antigen in the skin, T$_{reg}$ cells greatly increase in number, begin to express activation markers (some of which, such as CTLA-4, are mediators of suppressive function), become potent suppressors, and progressively accumulate in the target tissue (the skin). Our results are consistent with findings that two major populations of Foxp3$^+$ T$_{reg}$ cells exist in human peripheral blood, which have been called "resting" T$_{reg}$ cells and "activated" T$_{reg}$ cells.[13] Resting T$_{reg}$ cells are recently derived from the thymus, express low levels of CTLA-4, are not actively cycling, and are inferior suppressors compared to activated T$_{reg}$ cells. In contrast, activated T$_{reg}$ cells are constitutively cycling, express higher levels of Foxp3 and CTLA-4, and are more potent suppressors.

If antigen expression in the skin is extinguished, some of these activated T$_{reg}$ cells persist in the tissue and continue to inhibit subsequent responses to the antigen. These long-surviving T$_{reg}$ cells fulfill the main criteria of memory cells, namely they are antigen experienced and have an activated phenotype, they survive without antigen in nonlymphoid tissues, and they show enhanced function. Our finding regarding memory T$_{reg}$ cells has been reproduced in the setting of pregnancy, in which maternal T$_{reg}$ cells specific for fetal antigens accumulate during pregnancy and persist following parturition. These memory T$_{reg}$ cells reaccumulate during subsequent pregnancies and promote the acceptance of the fetal graft.[14]

These results make the key point that the life history of T$_{reg}$ cells is fundamentally similar to that of other (conventional) T cells (Fig. 1). Both are naive when they complete their maturation in the thymus and emerge to populate peripheral lymphoid tissues. They acquire effector function only after they encounter antigen, subsequently expand and migrate to the target tissue, and a fraction survives as memory cells. Thus, the sequence of naive to effector to memory may be characteristic of all lymphocytes, certainly in the T cell lineage. Needless to say, there are likely important differences in the signals that drive conventional T cells and T$_{reg}$ cells through these sequential stages.

Peripheral T$_{reg}$ cells

We have studied the generation of pT$_{reg}$ cells by transferring antigen-specific CD4$^+$ T cells into mice expressing the cognate antigen as a circulating systemic protein.[15] These experiments have established that in response to antigen, naive T cells first develop into pathogenic effector cells that cause inflammatory disease. In a subsequent wave of differentiation, pT$_{reg}$ cells develop with a slight delay compared to effector T cells and eventually mediate resolution of the inflammatory disease (Fig. 2). The thymus is dispensable for this process. The same sequence has been observed in similar studies of responses to cutaneous antigen, as has the persistence of T$_{reg}$ cells as memory cells.[16] Thus, the life history of peripheral T$_{reg}$ cells is likely much the same as that of thymic T$_{reg}$ cells, following the sequence of naive to effector to memory.

Signals for the generation and maintenance of T$_{reg}$ cells

The realization of the role of T$_{reg}$ cells in preventing autoimmunity, and the potential of therapies based

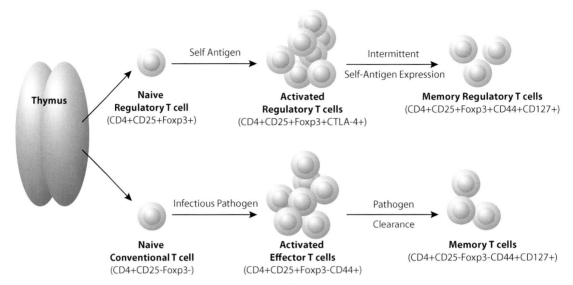

Figure 1. Stages in the lives of conventional and regulatory T cells. Both tT_{reg} cells and conventional T cells are naive when they complete their maturation in the thymus and emerge to populate peripheral lymphoid tissues. They become activated, expand, and acquire effector function after encountering antigen (presumably tissue self-antigen or commensal microbiota for T_{reg} cells, and microbial pathogens for conventional T cells). A fraction of antigen-experienced cells survive as memory cells. T_{reg} cells parallel conventional T cells in the sequential development from naive to effector to memory cells.

on T_{reg} cell transfer or activation, have led to many efforts to define the signals that are responsible for generating and maintaining these cells. Our own studies have focused on two sets of signals—the cytokine interleukin-2 (IL-2) and antigen itself.

Interleukin 2

The discovery that knockout of the gene for IL-2 or either the α or β chain of the IL-2 receptor results not in immune deficiency but in systemic autoimmunity has radically changed our understanding of the function of IL-2. It is now accepted that the main, nonredundant role of IL-2 is the maintenance of functional T_{reg} cells.[17] We have shown that IL-2 is required for the survival of T_{reg} and also for their functional competence.[18] The cytokine likely maintains T_{reg} cell function by promoting expression of Foxp3 and mediators of suppression, notably CTLA-4.

The experimental models we have established are unique in that effector and regulatory T cells are induced sequentially *in vivo* by the same antigen, allowing us to explore the role of signals such as IL-2 in the development of both cell populations. We now know that the disease induced by transfer of IL-2–deficient T cells into antigen-expressing mice is less severe and delayed compared to disease caused

by IL-2 competent wild-type T cells. This is likely due to reduced survival and/or expansion of effector cells.[15] However, the disease does develop, showing that pathogenic effector cells can be generated even in the absence of this key T cell growth factor. In contrast, the disease does not resolve in the absence of IL-2, because of a failure of T_{reg} cell generation. These results have led to the conclusion that IL-2 promotes the development of effector T cells (especially Th1 cells in models of tissue inflammation) and is essential for the generation and function of T_{reg} cells (Fig. 2). This revision of our view of the functions of IL-2 is the basis for recent, small clinical trials examining the ability of low-dose IL-2 administration to treat inflammatory diseases.[19,20]

Finally, a puzzle in the field has been that T_{reg} cells require IL-2 for peripheral generation as well as for function but do not themselves produce the cytokine. What, then, is the source of IL-2 for induction and maturation of T_{reg} cells? Our results suggest that IL-2 made during conventional immune responses to foreign antigens (e.g., microbes) acts first on Foxp3+ T cells in the tissues.[21] Thus, responses to environmental antigens may provide enough IL-2 to maintain a full T_{reg} cell repertoire in healthy individuals. This dependence of T_{reg} cells on IL-2, which they cannot produce themselves but

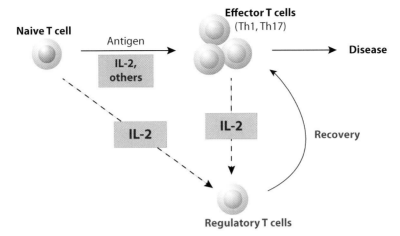

Figure 2. Sequential development of effector and regulatory T cells. Autoreactive T cells that respond to their cognate antigen become activated and develop into effector cells and cause autoimmune disease. Recovery from this disease is associated with the subsequent generation of FoxP3$^+$ CD25$^+$ regulatory cells in the periphery. Both pathogenic effector cells and protective regulatory cells develop from the same antigen-specific T cell population after activation, and their generation may occur in parallel or sequentially. IL-2 plays a dual role in this systemic T cell reaction. Upon antigen contact, effector T cells produce IL-2, which not only supports the expansion and survival of effector T cells but also is most importantly an essential factor for the development of pT$_{reg}$ cells. These peripheral T$_{reg}$ cells can then suppress the effector response and lead to resolution of disease, a process that does not occur in the absence of IL-2.

instead receive from conventional T cells, provides a very elegant negative feedback loop through which the ratio between T$_{reg}$ cells and conventional T cells is controlled.

Antigen

We have also explored the role of antigen in the development of effector and regulatory T cells. Preliminary studies have shown that persistent antigen expression, which mimics self-antigen, eliminates effector cells, and maintains T$_{reg}$ cells, whereas transient antigen exposure (resembling an infection) does the opposite.[16] Such systems provide an opportunity to explore the biochemical pathways triggered by antigen recognition in effector and regulatory T cells.

Future studies

The discovery of memory T$_{reg}$ cells has relied on transgenic mouse models in which a population with a single TCR of defined specificity can be followed quantitatively. An important priority is to determine if the same differentiation pathway is seen in polyclonal populations in response to self-antigen. However, TCR-transgenic models will remain a valuable tool for elucidating the conditions required for formation and maintenance of memory T$_{reg}$ cells. The results will subsequently have

to be confirmed in clinical settings. Peripheral T$_{reg}$ cell generation is typically studied by us and others in lymphopenic hosts, and following these cells in recipients with intact immune systems is also an important goal. Finally, we have begun to ask if similar T$_{reg}$ cell populations can be defined and analyzed in humans. Remarkably, on the basis of initial studies, memory T$_{reg}$ cells seem to be abundant in normal human skin. The development and maintenance of memory T$_{reg}$ cells may be important in multiple settings, such as relapsing–remitting autoimmune conditions, the maternal–fetal conflict in pregnancy, and potentially even recurring cancer, where the preservation of T$_{reg}$ cells specific for altered self would increase the risk of recurrence. Therefore, understanding the generation and maintenance of memory T$_{reg}$ cells in humans is an important future goal.

Conflicts of interest

The authors declare no conflicts of interest.

References

1. Bluestone, J.A. & A.K. Abbas. 2003. Natural versus adaptive regulatory T cells. *Nat. Rev. Immunol.* **3:** 253–257.
2. Lathrop, S.K., S.M. Bloom, S.M. Rao, *et al.* 2011. Peripheral education of the immune system by colonic commensal microbiota. *Nature* **478:** 250–254.

3. Haribhai, D., W. Lin, B. Edwards, *et al.* 2009. A central role for induced regulatory T cells in tolerance induction in experimental colitis. *J. Immunol.* **182:** 3461–3468.

4. Feuerer, M., J.A. Hill, K. Kretschmer, *et al.* 2010. Genomic definition of multiple ex vivo regulatory T cell subphenotypes. *Proc. Natl. Acad. Sci. USA* **107:** 5919–5924.

5. Long, M., S.-G. Park, I. Strickland, *et al.* 2009. Nuclear factor-kappaB modulates regulatory T cell development by directly regulating expression of Foxp3 transcription factor. *Immunity* **31:** 921–931.

6. Sauer, S., L. Bruno, A. Hertweck, *et al.* 2008. T cell receptor signaling controls Foxp3 expression via PI3K, Akt, and mTOR. *Proc. Natl. Acad. Sci. USA* **105:** 7797–7802.

7. Haxhinasto, S., D. Mathis & C. Benoist. 2008. The AKT-mTOR axis regulates de novo differentiation of CD4+Foxp3+ cells. *J. Exp. Med.* **205:** 565–574.

8. Chang, C.-F., W.N. D'Souza, I.L. Ch'en, *et al.* 2012. Polar opposites: Erk direction of CD4 T cell subsets. *J. Immunol.* **189:** 721–731.

9. Willoughby, J.E., P.S. Costello, R.H. Nicolas, *et al.* 2007. Raf signaling but not the ERK effector SAP-1 is required for regulatory T cell development. *J. Immunol.* **179:** 6836–6844.

10. Curotto de Lafaille, M.A. & J.J. Lafaille. 2009. Natural and adaptive foxp3+ regulatory T cells: more of the same or a division of labor? *Immunity* **30:** 626–635.

11. Benoist, C. & D. Mathis. 2012. Treg cells, life history, and diversity. *Cold Spring Harb. Perspect. Biol.* **4:** a007021. doi: 10.1101/cshperspect.a007021.

12. Rosenblum, M.D., I.K. Gratz, J.S. Paw, *et al.* 2011. Response to self antigen imprints regulatory memory in tissues. *Nature* **480:** 538–542.

13. Miyara, M., Y. Yoshioka, A. Kitoh, *et al.* 2009. Functional delineation and differentiation dynamics of human CD4+ T cells expressing the FoxP3 transcription factor. *Immunity* **30:** 899–911.

14. Rowe, J.H., J.M. Ertelt, L. Xin & S.S. Way. 2012. Pregnancy imprints regulatory memory that sustains anergy to fetal antigen. *Nature* **490:** 102–106.

15. Knoechel, B., J. Lohr, E. Kahn, *et al.* 2005. Sequential development of interleukin 2-dependent effector and regulatory T cells in response to endogenous systemic antigen. *J. Exp. Med.* **202:** 1375–1386.

16. Gratz, I.K., M.D. Rosenblum, J.S. Paw, *et al.* Self-antigen controls the balance between effector and regulatory T cells in peripheral tissues. *Proc. Natl. Acad. Sci. USA*: submitted.

17. Malek, T.R. 2008. The biology of interleukin-2. *Annu. Rev. Immunol.* **26:** 453–479.

18. Barron, L., H. Dooms, K.K. Hoyer, *et al.* 2010. Cutting edge: mechanisms of IL-2-dependent maintenance of functional regulatory T cells. *J. Immunol.* **185:** 6426–6430.

19. Koreth, J., K. Matsuoka, H.T. Kim, *et al.* 2011. Interleukin-2 and regulatory T cells in graft-versus-host disease. *N. Engl. J. Med.* **365:** 2055–2066.

20. Saadoun, D., M. Rosenzwajg, F. Joly, *et al.* 2011. Regulatory T-cell responses to low-dose interleukin-2 in HCV-induced vasculitis. *N. Engl. J. Med.* **365:** 2067–2077.

21. O'Gorman, W.E., H. Dooms, S.H. Thorne, *et al.* 2009. The initial phase of an immune response functions to activate regulatory T cells. *J. Immunol.* **183:** 332–339.

Ann. N.Y. Acad. Sci. ISSN 0077-8923

ANNALS OF THE NEW YORK ACADEMY OF SCIENCES

Issue: *Translational Immunology in Asia-Oceania*

Cross-reactive humoral responses to influenza and their implications for a universal vaccine

Christopher Chiu,[1,2,4] Jens Wrammert,[1,2,3] Gui-Mei Li,[1,2] Megan McCausland,[1,2] Patrick C. Wilson,[5] and Rafi Ahmed[1,2]

[1]Emory Vaccine Center, [2]Department of Microbiology and Immunology, [3]Department of Pediatric Infectious Disease, Department of Hematology and Oncology, Emory University School of Medicine, Atlanta, Georgia. [4]Center for Respiratory Infection, National Heart and Lung Institute, Imperial College London, London, United Kingdom. [5]Department of Medicine, Section of Rheumatology, The Committee on Immunology, The Knapp Center for Lupus and Immunology Research, The University of Chicago, Chicago, Illinois

Address for correspondence: Rafi Ahmed, Emory Vaccine Center, Department of Microbiology and Immunology, Emory University School of Medicine, G211, 1510 Clifton Road, Atlanta, GA 30322. rahmed@emory.edu

Influenza remains one of the most important causes of respiratory infection despite the widespread availability of vaccines. As effective vaccines against influenza principally rely on the induction of strain-specific neutralizing antibodies for their protective efficacy, drifted escape mutants and genetically reassortant pandemic strains can rapidly overcome them. Several groups have recently described cross-reactive influenza antibodies in humans, some of which bind to the conserved hemagglutinin stem. If such antibodies could be consistently induced at high levels by vaccines, they might protect against both seasonal and pandemic influenza strains. Here we discuss the humoral responses to influenza infection and vaccination, with particular reference to the pandemic H1N1 2009 virus and induction of broadly cross-reactive stem-binding antibodies. Having shown that cross-reactive antibodies are preferentially induced by a pandemic hemagglutinin, the challenge is now to design a vaccine that applies these principles to the induction of heterosubtypic immunity.

Keywords: antibodies; B cells; vaccination; influenza; hemagglutinin; stem

Introduction

Despite continuing advances in our understanding of the immune response to influenza infection and vaccination, the disease remains one of the foremost causes of morbidity and mortality worldwide. In the United States alone, influenza causes around 36,000 deaths per annum[1] and is responsible for a massive economic burden, with the total cost of each winter influenza epidemic estimated at over US$87 billion.[2] One of the principal factors underlying influenza's ability to cause reinfection is the rapid on-going mutation of its surface antigenic determinants. Influenza A expresses two major surface glycoproteins, hemagglutinin (HA) and neuraminidase (NA), both of which are targets for humoral immunity.[3] HA allows viral attachment to sialic acid and causes membrane fusion within the endosome, allowing viral entry.[4] In contrast, NA functions at the other end of the viral life cycle by cleaving sialic acid to allow the virion to escape the host cell surface.[5] Antibodies that bind to HA, in particular, are able to prevent infection and therefore are the basis on which vaccines against influenza are formulated.[6]

HA is a polypeptide consisting of two major extracellular domains: a globular head (the HA1 subunit) and a stalk that links to the transmembrane region (HA2).[7] There are typically four to five main binding sites for neutralizing antibodies, and, until recently, it was believed that all neutralizing antibodies were directed against immunodominant epitopes in the head.[8–10] This domain contains the receptor binding site but also numerous variable regions that are responsible for the extensive sequence divergence between strains. Variation in these areas contributes to antigenic differences in the 16 HA

doi: 10.1111/nyas.12012

subtypes, which are then classified into 2 phylogenetic groups.[11,12] Group 1 contains pathogens such as H1 and H5, while group 2 contains H3. Under constant immune pressure by neutralizing antibodies, epitopes in the head region undergo cumulative amino acid substitutions, leading to the phenomenon of antigenic drift and the generation of escape mutants.[13] In addition, the segmented genome of influenza, multiple animal reservoirs, and potential for coinfections with more than one influenza strain means that genome reassortment can occur, leading to antigenic shift.[14] While antigenic drift is responsible for recurrent seasonal epidemics, antigen shift can lead to the wholesale introduction of HA and NA variants to which large sections of the population have no immunity, thereby causing pandemics. The most recent of these started in 2009 with a swine-originated H1N1 virus;[15] and the potential still remains for a devastating pandemic to occur with a variant of a highly pathogenic avian H5N1 circulating primarily in Southeast Asia.[16]

Vaccines against influenza currently rely on the generation of neutralizing antibodies against HA and, to a lesser extent, NA.[6] These are highly strain specific, such that seasonal influenza vaccines must contain HAs from both H1 and H3 subtypes as well as influenza B, all matched to the prevailing strains in circulation.[17] Furthermore, both the inactivated and live attenuated vaccines provide only short-lived protection against the strains predicted to be circulating during each winter season.[18] Even in the absence of mutation, the half-life of neutralizing antibodies stimulated by vaccination can be around seven months, indicating a rapid waning of protective responses.[19] Annual revaccination is therefore necessary. In years where the vaccine strains are well matched to the circulating viruses, efficacy can reach 80% although this can be as little as 40% in the elderly population.[17,20,21] When circulating strains have already drifted or shifted significantly by the time the vaccine is finalized, vaccine efficacy is poor. Since the process of producing and testing vaccines is time consuming, the emergence of new strains is met by a substantial delay before suitable vaccines become available. No influenza vaccine has yet been developed to overcome these problems by eliciting protection against evolving virus strains. Thus, a "universal" vaccine that elicits durable and broadly protective immunity remains elusive. Further understanding of the humoral response to vaccination and infection with influenza is essential for achieving that goal.

The humoral response to the seasonal trivalent inactivated influenza vaccine

Our recent work has provided a detailed analysis of the events that occur after vaccination, both clarifying the mechanisms of action of influenza vaccines and developing tools that have highlighted potential avenues for their improvement. We first showed that healthy individuals, following receipt of the seasonal trivalent inactivated influenza vaccine (TIV), mounted a transient plasmablast response that peaked around day 7 post-vaccination and returned to baseline levels by day 14 (Fig. 1A and B).[22,23] The average peak frequency of these plasmablasts was around 6.4% of total B cells by flow cytometric analysis and all had phenotypic evidence of recent activation and proliferation, as shown by high levels of HLA-DR and Ki-67 expression (Fig. 1C). The size of the plasmablast burst correlated with fold change in hemagglutination inhibition titer, indicating that these cells were acutely responsible for the production of neutralizing antibody (Fig. 1D).

ELISPOT analysis of plasmablasts isolated by flow cytometric cell sorting revealed that the majority were influenza specific (average 70%). They were also mainly class-switched IgG-producing cells, suggesting that they were derived from the memory B cell compartment. We proceeded to examine the breadth of the immunoglobulin repertoire generated by these plasmablasts. This was achieved by sorting of single plasmablasts at the peak of the post-vaccination response, followed by RT-PCR of the heavy and light variable regions and then cloning of these products into expression vectors to generate recombinant monoclonal antibodies (mAbs). The results of this showed that a large proportion of the plasmablast population arose from relatively few clones. In our analysis, 61% of mAbs bound to the influenza strains contained in the vaccine and 60% of those were specific for HA. These mAbs were of high affinity and showed evidence of extensive somatic hypermutation, which, together with the speed of the response, suggested that they were the products of memory B cell differentiation.

Using these techniques, we therefore demonstrated the rapid recall response induced by

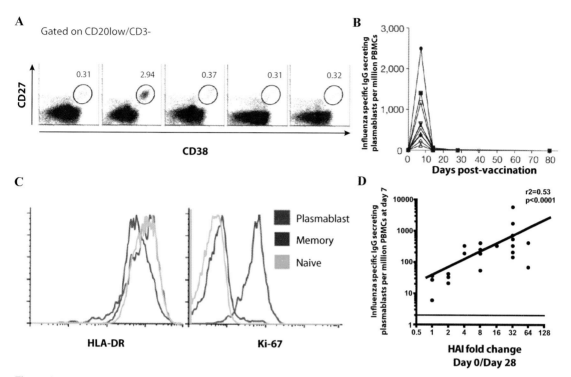

Figure 1. Influenza vaccination induces short-lived plasmablast proliferation that correlates with seroconversion. (A) Plasmablasts were analyzed in blood by flow cytometry, gating on $CD3^-CD20^{-/low}CD27^{hi}CD38^{hi}$ cells. Plots are shown at time points up to 28 days in a representative donor. (B) Influenza-specific plasmablasts were enumerated by ELISPOT using PBMCs from 10 donors at time points up to 80 days post-vaccination. Samples were assayed in duplicate and the mean plotted as plasmablasts per million PBMCs. (C) Plasmablasts at the peak of response (day 7 post-vaccination) were costained with HLA-DR or Ki-67 and compared with naive and memory B cells. A representative flow cytometric analysis is shown. (D) Twenty-four healthy adults were vaccinated with the pandemic H1N1 2009 vaccine. The number of vaccine-specific IgG-producing plasmablasts at the peak of response in 24 patients was correlated with fold change in hemagglutination inhibition titer between 0 and 28 days post-vaccination by Spearman's correlation. This figure was adapted from Refs. 22 and 33.

TIV and developed a method for quickly generating high affinity mAbs against influenza.

Broadly cross-reactive stem-binding antibodies dominate the response to H1N1 2009 pandemic influenza infection

In April 2009, a novel influenza strain emerged that was first reported in Mexico and appeared to have a reassortant genome derived from swine, avian, and human viruses.[15] This virus spread rapidly and the first pandemic of the 21st century was declared two months later. Because this pandemic strain was antigenically distinct from preceding seasonal strains it was believed that large segments of the population possessed little or no immunity to it.[14] This was particularly true of the young adult age groups who were disproportionately affected.

During the 2009 pandemic, we recruited nine patients with PCR-confirmed pandemic H1N1 2009 infection.[24] They presented with a spectrum of disease severity; most exhibited only mild short-lived symptoms with rapid viral clearance but two required hospitalization. One of the latter suffered respiratory failure and underwent mechanical ventilation with a prolonged in-patient stay. Over half of the others were treated with NA inhibitors, and samples were collected between 9 and 31 days after symptom onset. All patients had detectable serum antibody titers against pandemic H1N1 at the time of sample collection.

Although the exact timing of inoculation was unknown, it was possible to observe influenza-specific plasmablasts in all infected patients at the time of sample collection, including later time points at which samples were obtained from the more

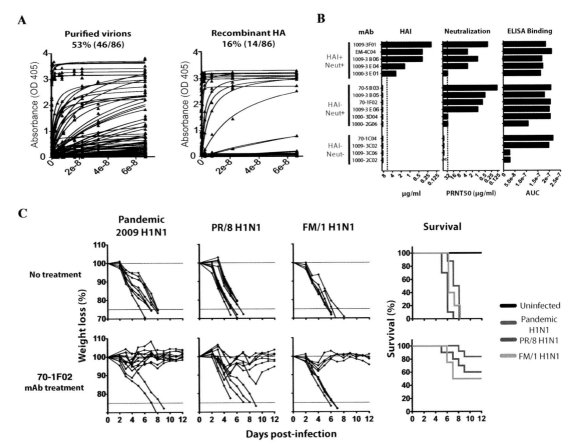

Figure 2. Broadly cross-reactive stem-binding antibodies against pandemic H1N1 2009 influenza virus from infected patients. Plasmablasts were sorted by flow cytometry at day 7 post-vaccination. Single plasmablasts were isolated and immunoglobulin variable genes cloned. (A) Scatchard binding plots show the binding of 86 individual monoclonal antibodies to the whole pandemic H1N1 2009 influenza virus (left panel) and to recombinant hemagglutinin from pandemic H1N1 2009 (right panel) by ELISA. (B) Hemagglutinin-specific monoclonal antibodies generated from single plasmablasts sorted from pandemic H1N1-infected patients were analyzed for binding and neutralizing capacity by hemagglutination inhibition, neutralization assay, and ELISA. HAI minimum effective antibody concentration, PRNT50 plaque reduction neutralization minimum effective antibody concentration, and minimum positive concentration for ELISA binding are shown. Assays were carried out in duplicate and repeated a minimum of three times. (C) Six- to eight-week-old BALB/c mice were treated with 200 μg of the stem-reactive monoclonal antibody 70–1F02 by intraperitoneal injection. After 12 hours, they were infected with 2 × LD_{50} of mouse-adapted pandemic H1N1, PR/8/34, or FM/1/47 virus. Daily body weight measurements and survival curves are shown. At least three repeat experiments were performed, and data from one representative experiment are shown. This figure was adapted from Ref. 24.

severely ill individuals. This suggested that virus-specific plasmablasts were present throughout infection due to the on-going presence of antigen. As with the vaccine-induced response, the majority of the cells were class-switched IgG-producing cells, and HA-specific cells accounted for up to 50% of virus-specific plasmablasts.

Interestingly, despite the known sequence divergence between the pandemic H1N12009HA and that of recent seasonal strains, most patients also had detectable plasmablast responses to HA from the seasonal influenza vaccine of that year. The presence of plasmablasts that reacted against the seasonal vaccine suggested that the pandemic H1N1 2009 virus might have induced cross-reactive responses. When 86 mAbs were cloned from sorted plasmablasts, 53% were virus specific, and around a third of those were directed against HA (Fig. 2A). Furthermore, analysis of their ability to bind to H1N1 strains from the three most recent seasonal influenza vaccines showed that the majority of HA-specific mAbs were cross-reactive.

Cross-reactive antibodies are directed against epitopes that are conserved between strains. These are most likely to exist within areas of structural importance, such as the receptor binding site. Here, amino acid changes lead to alterations in the essential functions of the protein and a fitness cost. Unsurprisingly, since the stem region of HA is required for membrane fusion, it is also highly conserved. Okuno *et al.* first reported broadly cross-reactive antibodies directed against this region in a mouse model infected with H2N2 in the 1990s.[25] The mAb described had no hemagglutination inhibition (HI) activity but was able to neutralize virus infection of cells *in vitro*, probably by blocking membrane fusion. This antibody could also confer protection from fatal infection by H1, H2, and H5 viruses in mice. Similar antibodies have only recently been recognized in humans as a result of novel high-throughput methods of mAb generation. Using phage display libraries[26–28] or immortalization of memory B cells in individuals previously vaccinated or infected with seasonal influenza A,[29] several groups have been able to clone broadly cross-reactive stem-binding antibodies. These reportedly share the V_H1–69 gene rearrangement and bind to a common region of the HA stem just below the head. One of these antibodies has recently been described to not only bind influenza A but also both lineages of influenza B.[30] Although direct estimates of the frequency of these stem-binding antibodies were not possible due to the B cell selection techniques used, it was clear that they were rare. The laborious screening of memory B cells for specificity against this region, for example, showed how infrequent they normally are.[29] This is most likely to be due to steric hindrance, as the trimeric HA molecules packed tightly on the surface of the virion interfere with B cell receptor recognition.[31,32]

Following infection with the pandemic H1N1 2009 influenza, we were surprised to find that mAbs with the characteristics of broadly cross-reactive stem binders were not only easily detected but also even dominated the response in some individuals. Overall, they made up over a third of HA-specific mAbs cloned from these patients. In common with stem-binding antibodies described elsewhere, these mAbs were able to bind to HA in ELISA assays and neutralized infection *in vitro* but did not inhibit hemagglutination of red blood cells by HI (Fig. 2B). Epitope mapping revealed that these mAbs were

indeed specific for an epitope in the stem region. They also shared the V_H1–69 gene rearrangement, and prophylactic treatment of mice confirmed that they were protective against weight loss and death from not only the pandemic H1N1 2009 strain but also the mouse adapted PR8 and the Fort Monmouth/1/1947 viruses (Fig. 2C).

The fact that mAbs specific for the pandemic H1N1 2009 virus were primarily class switched and showed extensive affinity maturation again implied that they were derived from plasmablasts generated through the proliferation of memory B cells. This was despite the fact that the HA from the pandemic strain diverged significantly from the most recent seasonal strains. We therefore analyzed PBMCs collected in 2008 to determine whether memory B cells that could recognize it were present prior to the emergence of the novel pandemic strain. The results showed that these memory B cells did already exist in spite of the fact that there was no possibility of the individuals having been exposed to pandemic H1N1 2009 HA. Together, these data indicated that the high frequency of stem-binding antibodies following pandemic H1N1 2009 infection resulted from the proliferation of cross-reactive memory B cells generated by prior exposure to divergent seasonal strains.

Can influenza vaccination induce broadly cross-reactive stem-binding antibodies?

From our data and other data, it was clear that the seasonal influenza vaccine does not normally induce stem-binding antibodies at easily detectable frequencies. In contrast, cross-reactive antibodies dominated the humoral response to pandemic H1N1 2009 infection, and a high proportion of them recognized the stem. A universal vaccine capable of inducing these broadly cross-reactive stem-binding antibodies at high frequency could provide the heterosubtypic immunity required to eradicate the need for annual revaccination. The first question was, therefore, whether a vaccine could induce these antibodies?

We hypothesized that the high frequency of stem-binding antibodies following pandemic H1N1 2009 infection was in part due to the differences in antigenicity of the novel HA and therefore could be replicated by vaccination. We therefore recruited 24 healthy adults vaccinated with a monovalent pandemic H1N1 2009 inactivated vaccine.[33] These

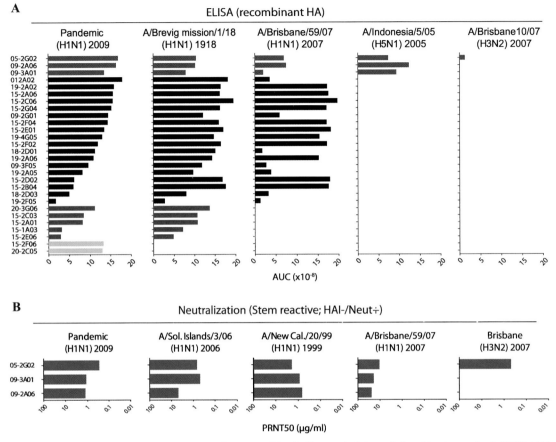

Figure 3. Cross-reactive antibodies against both the stem and head of hemagglutinin are induced by the pandemic H1N1 2009 vaccine. Monoclonal antibodies were generated from single plasmablasts sorted at day 7 post-vaccination from eight pandemic H1N1 2009 vaccines. (A) Monoclonal antibodies were assayed for binding by ELISA to recombinant hemagglutinins from influenza A/California/4/2009, A/Brevig Mission/1/1918, A/Brisbane/59/2007, A/Indonesia/5/2005 (H5N1), and A/Brisbane/10/2007 (H3N2). Antibodies are placed in four groups according to the degree of binding by ELISA to the pandemic H1N1 2009 HA and the degree of cross-reactivity, with blue = high cross-reactivity, black and red = intermediate cross-reactivity, and green = no cross-reactivity. (B) Three stem-binding antibodies were assayed for neutralizing activity against a panel of influenza virus strains with increasing divergence from the pandemic H1N1 2009 virus, from left to right. Data are representative of two to four repeat experiments. This figure was adapted from Ref. 33.

individuals were enrolled around six months after the emergence of the pandemic strain and were given the monovalent vaccine separately from the seasonal TIV. Similar to the response to seasonal TIV, the monovalent pandemic H1N1 2009 vaccine induced a rapid plasmablast response that peaked at around day 7 and was primarily composed of IgG-producing cells. Monoclonal antibodies were generated from eight individuals and about 58% of them bound to the pandemic H1N1 2009 virus. Of these, 62% were HA-specific by ELISA.

As predicted, the shared antigenic properties of the vaccine led to a breadth of antibody response that was, in many ways, similar to that following infection. The majority of mAbs were cross-reactive, able to bind and neutralize most or all recent seasonal influenza strains in addition to the homologous pandemic H1N1 2009 strain (Fig. 3A). In addition, three mAbs were stem binding. These displayed increased cross-reactivity, with evidence of heterosubtypic binding to a H5N1 HA (Fig. 3A and B). One of these displayed an even greater breadth, neutralizing viruses across both phylogenetic groups 1 (H1N1) and 2 (H3N2) despite their significant sequence divergence. Extremely cross-reactive stembinding antibodies, such as the above, and the mAb

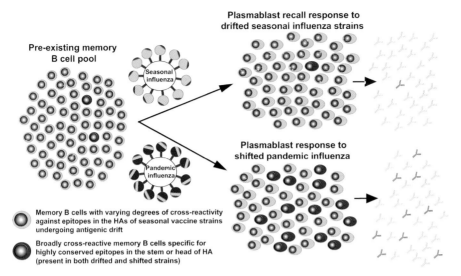

Figure 4. The antibody response following exposure to seasonal versus pandemic influenza virus strains. All adults have a pool of preexisting influenza-specific memory B cells, most of which recognize epitopes from the HA head from recent seasonal strains (shown in green). These change relatively little year to year due to antigenic drift, so the same memory B cells are repeatedly expanded by infection or vaccination and come to dominate the repertoire. Memory B cells that recognize highly conserved epitopes in the head and stem (shown in red) therefore remain in the minority. However, when a pandemic strain emerges, most of those previously immunodominant epitopes in the HA head are replaced (shown in blue), leaving only the conserved epitopes in the stem and head. Cross-reactive memory B cells specific for these epitopes are therefore rapidly recruited into the response and come to dominate it. Naive responses to the novel epitopes in the head are primed more slowly and therefore make a relatively small contribution to the new response. This figure was adapted from Ref. 33.

described by Corti *et al.* that binds all 16 HA subtypes prove that a truly universal heterosubtypic humoral response can be induced.[34] We have also shown that even an inactivated vaccine with no adjuvant can stimulate this type of response.[33]

Assuming a universal response can be induced, however, why are cross-reactive antibodies not commonly found in the population? We believe that broadly cross-reactive antibodies are produced by low-frequency memory B cells reactive against conserved but subdominant epitopes (Fig. 4). These epitopes are most highly conserved in the HA stem but also occur in the head. In the context of seasonal influenza, these have a low probability of being recruited into the response and thus remain quiescent due to competition by the more numerous B cells specific for immunodominant epitopes present in the globular HA head. For this reason, such antibodies are rare in most individuals. However, following antigenic shift, most immunodominant epitopes in the head are replaced with novel antibody binding sites. With the disappearance of immunodominant epitopes, only the subdominant conserved epitopes shared between seasonal and pandemic strains are

present to stimulate cross-reactive memory B cells. These then have the opportunity to differentiate and proliferate more quickly than naive B cells primed by novel epitopes. Cross-reactive antibodies therefore make up a greater proportion of the humoral immune response with a pandemic strain, whether in the context of infection or vaccination.

However, the number of stem-binding mAbs remains relatively small following pandemic H1N1 2009 vaccination, and they are not readily found in every vaccinee. This contrasts with the abundant stem-binding antibody responses seen following natural infection.[24] There may be several explanations for this. Since viral subunits cannot infect cells they are subject to extrinsic antigen presentation pathways;[35] they also induce less potent inflammatory and innate responses. Conversely, infection results in greater antigen load and duration, leading to increased recruitment of precursors and signals for differentiation.[36] A novel heterosubtypic vaccine must therefore overcome these issues and elicit a response that is similar to or even greater than the response to natural infection. Whether this is best achieved using novel antigenic constructs,[37] adjuvants,[38] or methods of delivery is under investigation.

Our recent data regarding the induction of highly cross-reactive stem-binding antibodies and the mechanisms by which they may be promoted have raised the prospects of a universal influenza vaccine. However, no vaccine yet exists that can induce the high frequencies of cross-reactive antibodies in all vaccinees required for robust cross-reactive immunity. The on-going challenge therefore remains to develop novel vaccines that elicit protective mechanisms beyond antibodies directed against the HA head at levels that provide long-lasting heterosubtypic protection.

Acknowledgments

This work was funded in part by National Institutes of Health (NIH)/National Institute of Allergy and Infectious Diseases (NIAID) Grant U19-AI057266 with American Recovery and Reinvestment Act Supplement U19 AI057266-06S2 (to R.A. and P.C.W.); NIH/NIAID Awards HHSN266200700006C Center of Excellence for Influenza Research and Surveillance (to R.A. and P.C.W.); HHSN266200500026C (to P.C.W.); and 5U19AI062629-05 (to P.C.W.).

Conflict of interest

R.A., J.W., and P.C.W. have a licensing agreement with MedImmune on the influenza virus–specific human monoclonal antibodies.

References

1. Thompson, W. *et al.* 2003. Mortality associated with influenza and respiratory syncytial virus in the United States. *JAMA* **289:** 179–186.
2. Molinari, N.A. *et al.* 2007. The annual impact of seasonal influenza in the US: measuring disease burden and costs. *Vaccine* **25:** 5086–5096.
3. Fields, B.N., D.M. Knipe & P.M. Howley. 2007. *Fields' Virology*. Wolters Kluwer/Lippincott Williams & Wilkins: Philadelphia, PA, London.
4. Skehel, J.J. & D.C. Wiley. 2000. Receptor binding and membrane fusion in virus entry: the influenza hemagglutinin. *Annu. Rev. Biochem.* **69:** 531–569.
5. Mitnaul, L.J. *et al.* 2000. Balanced hemagglutinin and neuraminidase activities are critical for efficient replication of influenza A virus. *J. Virol.* **74:** 6015–6020.
6. Ellebedy, A.H. & R.J. Webby. 2009. Influenza vaccines. *Vaccine* **27:** D65–D68.
7. Ward, C.W. 1981. Structure of the influenza virus hemagglutinin. *Curr. Top. Microbiol. Immunol.* **94–95:** 1–74.
8. Caton, A.J., G.G. Brownlee, J.W. Yewdell & W. Gerhard. 1982. The antigenic structure of the influenza virus A/PR/8/34 hemagglutinin (H1 subtype). *Cell* **31:** 417–427.
9. Wiley, D.C., I.A. Wilson & J.J. Skehel. 1981. Structural identification of the antibody-binding sites of Hong Kong influenza haemagglutinin and their involvement in antigenic variation. *Nature* **289:** 373–378.
10. Wilson, I.A. & N.J. Cox. 1990. Structural basis of immune recognition of influenza virus hemagglutinin. *Annu. Rev. Immunol.* **8:** 737–787.
11. Nabel, G.J. & A.S. Fauci. 2010. Induction of unnatural immunity: prospects for a broadly protective universal influenza vaccine. *Nat. Med.* **16:** 1389–1391.
12. Sui, J. *et al.* 2011. Wide prevalence of heterosubtypic broadly neutralizing human anti-influenza A antibodies. *Clin Infect Dis.* **52:** 1003–1009.
13. Yewdell, J.W., R.G. Webster & W.U. Gerhard. 1979. Antigenic variation in three distinct determinants of an influenza type A haemagglutinin molecule. *Nature* **279:** 246–248.
14. Garten, R.J. *et al.* 2009. Antigenic and genetic characteristics of swine-origin 2009 A(H1N1) influenza viruses circulating in humans. *Science* **325:** 197–201.
15. Novel Swine-Origin Influenza A (H1N1) Virus Investigation Team *et al.* 2009. Emergence of a novel swine-origin influenza A (H1N1) virus in humans. *N. Engl. J. Med.* **360:** 2605–2615.
16. Subbarao, K. *et al.* 1998. Characterization of an avian influenza A (H5N1) virus isolated from a child with a fatal respiratory illness. *Science* **279:** 393–396.
17. Osterholm, M.T., N.S. Kelley, A. Sommer & E.A. Belongia. 2012. Efficacy and effectiveness of influenza vaccines: a systematic review and meta-analysis. *Lancet Infect. Dis.* **12:** 36–44.
18. Ambrose, C.S., M.J. Levin & R.B. Belshe. 2011. The relative efficacy of trivalent live attenuated and inactivated influenza vaccines in children and adults. *Influenza Other Respir. Viruses* **5:** 67–75.
19. Wright, P.F. *et al.* 2008. Antibody responses after inactivated influenza vaccine in young children. *Pediatr. Infect. Dis. J.* **27:** 1004–1008.
20. Hannoun, C., F. Megas & J. Piercy. 2004. Immunogenicity and protective efficacy of influenza vaccination. *Virus Res.* **103:** 133–138.
21. Monto, A.S. *et al.* 2009. Comparative efficacy of inactivated and live attenuated influenza vaccines. *N. Engl. J. Med.* **361:** 1260–1267.
22. Wrammert, J. *et al.* 2008. Rapid cloning of high-affinity human monoclonal antibodies against influenza virus. *Nature* **453:** 667–671.
23. Smith, K. *et al.* 2009. Rapid generation of fully human monoclonal antibodies specific to a vaccinating antigen. *Nature Protocols* **4:** 372–384.
24. Wrammert, J. *et al.* 2011. Broadly cross-reactive antibodies dominate the human B cell response against 2009 pandemic H1N1 influenza virus infection. *J. Exp. Med.* **208:** 181.
25. Okuno, Y., Y. Isegawa, F. Sasao & S. Ueda. 1993. A common neutralizing epitope conserved between the hemagglutinins of influenza A virus H1 and H2 strains. *J. Virol.* **67:** 2552–2558.
26. Throsby, M. *et al.* 2008. Heterosubtypic neutralizing monoclonal antibodies cross-protective against H5N1 and H1N1 recovered from human IgM+ memory B cells. *PLoS One* **3:** e3942.

27. Ekiert, D.C. *et al.* 2009. Antibody recognition of a highly conserved influenza virus epitope. *Science* **324:** 246–251.

28. Sui, J. *et al.* 2009. Structural and functional bases for broad-spectrum neutralization of avian and human influenza A viruses. *Nat. Struct. Mol. Biol.* **16:** 265–273.

29. Corti, D. *et al.* 2010. Heterosubtypic neutralizing antibodies are produced by individuals immunized with a seasonal influenza vaccine. *J. Clin. Invest.* **120:** 1663–1673.

30. Dreyfus, C. *et al.* 2012. Highly conserved protective epitopes on influenza B viruses. *Science* **337:** 1343–1348.

31. Calder, L.J., S. Wasilewski, J.A. Berriman & P.B. Rosenthal. 2010. Structural organization of a filamentous influenza A virus. *Proc. Natl. Acad. Sci. USA* **107:** 10685–10690.

32. Harris, A. *et al.* 2006. Influenza virus pleiomorphy characterized by cryoelectron tomography. *Proc. Natl. Acad. Sci. USA* **103:** 19123–19127.

33. Li, G.-M. *et al.* 2012. Pandemic H1N1 influenza vaccine induces a recall response in humans that favors broadly cross-reactive memory B cells. *PNAS* **109:** 9047–9052.

34. Corti, D. *et al.* 2011. A neutralizing antibody selected from plasma cells that binds to group 1 and group 2 influenza A hemagglutinins. *Science* **333:** 850–856.

35. Sasaki, S. *et al.* 2006. Comparison of the influenza virus-specific effector and memory B-cell responses to immunization of children and adults with live attenuated or inactivated influenza virus vaccines. *J. Virol.* **81:** 215–228.

36. Kreijtz, J.H.C.M., R.A.M. Fouchier & G.F. Rimmelzwaan. 2011. Immune responses to influenza virus infection. *Virus Res.* **162:** 19–30.

37. Steel, J. *et al.* 2010. Influenza virus vaccine based on the conserved hemagglutinin stalk domain. *MBio* pii: e00018-10. doi: 10.1128/mBio.00018-10.

38. Khurana, S. *et al.* 2011. MF59 adjuvant enhances diversity and affinity of antibody-mediated immune response to pandemic influenza vaccines. *Sci. Transl. Med.* **3:** 85ra48.

Ann. N.Y. Acad. Sci. ISSN 0077-8923

ANNALS OF THE NEW YORK ACADEMY OF SCIENCES

Issue: *Translational Immunology in Asia-Oceania*

The dual role of biomarkers for understanding basic principles and devising novel intervention strategies in tuberculosis

January Weiner 3rd, Jeroen Maertzdorf, and Stefan H.E. Kaufmann

Max Planck Institute for Infection Biology, Department of Immunology, Berlin, Germany

Address for correspondence: Stefan H.E. Kaufmann, Max Planck Institute for Infection Biology, Department of Immunology, Charitéplatz 1, 10117 Berlin, Germany. Kaufmann@mpiib-berlin.mpg.de

There is great need for better control measures for tuberculosis (TB). High-throughput analyses, such as transcriptomic and metabolic profiling, offer a promising path toward clinically useful biosignatures. With the help of biomarkers, it will be possible not only to reliably perform diagnosis but also to gain a better understanding of the disease process and, in the future, even predict the onset of disease in infected individuals. Biomarkers based on transcriptomic and metabolic profiles as well as on cytokine composition provide important insights into the basic biological principles of TB and give an opportunity to reliably distinguish TB patients from healthy individuals. Use of biomarkers for point-of-care diagnosis, however, is still a distant goal, which to achieve will require extensive analysis of TB biosignatures across different cohorts and a combination of different platforms.

Keywords: tuberculosis; biomarkers; transcriptomics; vaccination

Introduction

Tuberculosis (TB) is a global health threat that annually afflicts about 9 million individuals, leading to some 1.5 million deaths.[1] Yet, it is not equally distributed worldwide.[2] Developing countries in Africa and Southeast Asia suffer most from this scourge. Most cases, however, occur in two countries in economic transition—India and China. The burden faced by India alone includes more than 3 million people with TB—with approximately 2.3 million new cases annually—of whom more than 10% will die.[1] To many people in the industrialized world these figures may come as a surprise. After all, since the 1960s, effective drugs have been in clinical use that cure TB, and a vaccine has been available for almost 100 years.[2] Unfortunately, all of these achievements supported by taxpayers and philanthropists of the past have largely lost their value today. In particular, decades of poor compliance to drug treatment has allowed the tubercle bacilli to develop drug resistance. Today, we are facing an increasing threat of multidrug-resistant (MDR) TB, as well as even extensively drug-resistant (XDR) TB and even totally drug-resistant (TDR) TB, which are difficult or virtually impossible to treat.[3] In India alone some 45,000 individuals develop MDR-TB every year,[1] and XDR-TB cases are on the rise. Moreover, the vaccine Bacille Calmette–Guérin (BCG) never fulfilled original expectations. Although it can prevent serious forms of TB in newborn infants, it is virtually ineffective against the most prevalent form of the disease today: pulmonary TB in adolescents and adults. Finally, diagnosis—which looks back on a history of 130 years—fails today in half of all cases. Most commonly, the diagnosis of TB targets the causative agent *Mycobacterium tuberculosis* (Mtb) in sputum smears using a test that is inexpensive but low in sensitivity—as low as 60% in some regions.[4] A more rapid and sensitive test is the recently developed GeneXpert® system[5] based on quantitative PCR, but which is prohibitively expensive, especially in regions with limited resources. Misdiagnosis of active TB results in treatment delays. As a corollary, a substantial number of untreated,

doi: 10.1111/j.1749-6632.2012.06802.x

Ann. N.Y. Acad. Sci. 1283 (2013) 22–29 © 2012 New York Academy of Sciences.

contagious patients promote continued transmission of TB.[6]

In the face of these cruel figures it may be surprising that in the vast majority of individuals infected with Mtb, disease will never develop, even though they remain infected for life.[7] These individuals with so-called latent TB infection (LTBI) harbor the pathogen but contain it by means of their immune response; hence, they are not contagious. The number of individuals with LTBI has been estimated to exceed 2 billion worldwide. Given that the distribution of individuals with LTBI is not uniform, that they are most prevalent in regions with high TB incidences, and that estimates of prevalence of individuals with LTBI in groups such as health-care workers reach almost 50%,[8] we assume that in many high-burden areas of India, a large proportion of adults are living with LTBI. However, because it is a dynamic process, 10% of all individuals with LTBI will develop the active disease during their lifetime.

Undoubtedly, better TB control based on novel intervention measures is needed.[4] Critical to the development of such measures are biomarkers that reliably diagnose or are prognostic of the disease and determine the response to intervention. We have embarked on the identification of biomarkers and the design of custom-made biosignatures that can ultimately fulfill the following criteria:

- reliably discriminate between active TB and health (either uninfected or with LTBI);
- better understand the mechanisms underlying infection, immunity, and pathogenesis; and
- predict risk of TB disease in individuals with LTBI.

The latter goal, although not yet accomplished, is particularly important for several reasons. First, prediction of disease risk can be used for stratification of study participants who are most prone to progress to active TB for inclusion in clinical trials, thus reducing both the numbers of participants and duration of such trials. Second, these biomarkers could help with monitoring clinical trials by serving as surrogate markers of intervention efficacy, which predict the clinical endpoint of active TB disease before clinical diagnosis. Conventional diagnostics classify disease status at a particular time point, whereas biomarkers can provide prognostic information, and thus reveal general mechanisms of disease pathogenesis.[9] In order to obtain robust prognostic information across different cohorts, it is imperative to direct our searches toward custom-made biosignatures comprising a selection of the best-suited markers rather than a single biomarker.[4,10] Such predictive biomarkers could help in the early identification of individuals with high risk of active TB so that they receive preventive drug treatment. Finally, the search for biomarkers using high-throughput (HT) platforms should not be restricted to pure statistical analysis of variables for classification purposes (Fig. 1). Rather, we argue that data evaluation should consider biological mechanisms underlying infection, immunity, and pathogenesis to develop an independent line of thought, which could ultimately lead to novel predictions and hypotheses.

Transcriptional biomarkers

Most of the early HT studies aimed at identifying new biomarkers in TB have used gene expression profiling in peripheral blood cells.[11–17] These studies provide a general picture of altered gene expression patterns in TB patients, most of which are indicative of persistent activation of the immune system in TB patients.

The most prominent gene expression signature in blood cells from TB patients is the elevated expression of upstream and downstream elements of the interferon signaling pathway, as pointed out by Berry *et al.*[14] and observed by others as well.[15,16] This increased activity in interferon signaling was shown to be most prominent in neutrophils in the peripheral blood. Among the most differentially expressed markers in TB are the Fc gamma receptors.[16] Further analysis also indicated that most response elements (i.e., downstream genes) in the Fc gamma receptor-mediated signaling pathway are affected in TB, indicating its central role in the pathology of this disease.[15]

The activation of the JAK-STAT pathway and increased expression of several elements therein, notably in T lymphocytes, was also identified in several studies.[14,15,18] Activation of this pathway correlates with increased cytokine expression and other immunological markers. Central regulators within this pathway are the suppressor of cytokine signaling (SOCS) molecules. One study related the differential expression of SOCS3 in T cells from TB patients and healthy controls to the regulation of cytokine

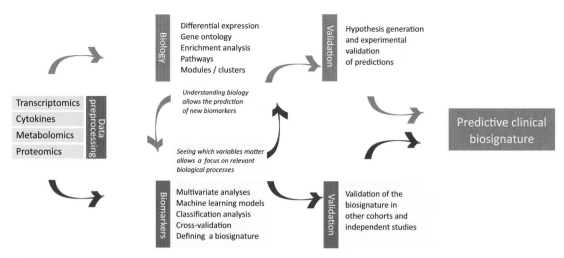

Figure 1. Understanding the biology underlying TB complements the search for biosignatures through experimental verification, novel hypotheses, and identification of new targets for research directions. Reciprocally, identification of specific and sensitive sets of biomarkers may unlock entry points for research. Together, these approaches will guide us toward a predictive biosignature.

signaling in T cells.[18] These analyses also identified a more general increase in the expression of innate defense response genes, including defensins, CEACAM cognates, complement factors, and Toll-like receptor (TLR) signaling molecules in TB patients.

For an extensive review of immunological markers, including cytokines/chemokines, membrane-bound and soluble receptors, and other inflammation markers, we refer the reader to a recent publication.[19] Since the most pronounced differences in gene expression between active TB and healthy controls suggest a chronic state of activation of the immune system in patients, immune markers and defense response genes have predictive potential for TB.[20]

Transcriptional biomarkers, though, need not be limited to analysis of expression of protein-coding genes. Gene expression is, in general, a tightly regulated and complex process, and changes in this process during infectious disease can be controlled at various levels. Furthermore, a much larger proportion of the human genome seems to be transcribed than previously assumed.[21] One major posttranscriptional level of regulation is controlled by microRNAs, small noncoding RNA molecules that target multiple gene transcripts.[22] HT analysis of microRNAs has been the focus of recent studies,[23–29] implicating several differentially expressed microRNAs in TB pathology and in the modulation of T cell cytokine and chemokine production in TB

patients. A recent analysis in murine TB revealed the central role of miR223 in control of neutrophil-driven inflammation.[30]

Although the discriminative signatures described in different studies vary in the magnitude of transcripts and numbers of genes, a common picture unfolds including type 1 interferon signaling, Fc gamma receptors, guanylate-binding proteins (GPBs), and defensins as major contributors. Thus, although gene expression can reliably distinguish between TB patients and healthy individuals, in our opinion, the implementation of a robust and inexpensive point-of-care test for diagnostic purposes still has a long way to go. As a first step toward this goal, validation of predictive signatures defined thus far in unique cohorts must be applied across diverse cohorts from different regions.

Differential gene expression between TB patients and healthy controls has been consistently identified in diverse cohorts. In contrast, differences between uninfected and LTBI individuals among healthy participants are generally less clear. Although some global gene expression profiling studies observed significant differences,[17,18] others did not.[14,15] Thus far only *ex vivo* stimulation of blood samples has resulted in differential expression levels of several cytokines between uninfected and LTBI individuals, although results between different studies are not uniform.[20] This issue, therefore, requires further investigation by different analytical platforms.

Metabolic profiling of infectious diseases

Metabolic profiling (also referred to as metabolomics or metabonomics) of serum or plasma monitors biological processes.[31] Metabolites are exchanged between tissues and organs through the blood, and hence metabolites measured in serum or plasma can derive from different organs. Furthermore, products from the microbiome, xenobiotic substances from the environment, and drugs and their metabolites are being measured. Finally, in the case of infectious diseases such as TB, metabolites from the etiologic agent(s) add to the complexity.

Thus far, metabolic profiling has been predominantly applied to cancer,[32] cardiovascular diseases,[33] and diabetes;[34] but changes in metabolic profiles are likely equally informative for infectious diseases such as TB. First, metabolic profiles can be expected to be influenced by environmental factors (such as malnourishment) or comorbidities, which lead to a higher risk of progressing to active TB (e.g., diabetes[35]). Second, inflammation—notably, nonresolving inflammation as in TB—is known for its general and systemic impact on host metabolism. Third, several metabolites, such as hormones including cortisol,[36] or intermediate metabolites, such as kynurenine, L-arginine,[37] and inosine,[38] are well-known signaling molecules of relevance to the immune response. Finally, metabolic profiling provides information complementary to transcriptome analysis with a different perspective on the biological processes active during disease.

Only few attempts have been made to understand the changes in metabolic profiles of the host during TB; however, a number of studies in other infectious diseases, notably pneumonia, illustrate marked metabolic alterations relevant to TB. Nuclear magnetic resonance (NMR)-based analysis of 61 metabolites in urine samples from adults suffering from community-acquired pneumonia[39] allowed the delineation of profiles characteristic for distinct forms of pneumonia caused by bacteria and viruses. Furthermore, biomarker profiles determined by mass spectrometry of matched plasma and urine samples allowed a robust differentiation of severe childhood pneumonia from healthy controls with an overall error rate below 15%.[40]

For TB, metabolic profiling has been performed with samples from experimental animals and patients. Metabolic profiling in serum, lung, spleen, and liver of mice infected with Mtb revealed differential abundances of 32 metabolites in uninfected and Mtb-infected mice, with the most profound differences in the lungs.[41] Intriguingly, differences in blood samples mirrored changes in the lung, suggesting that metabolic profiles in the peripheral blood reflect changes in the affected organ, at least partially. Several changes observed could be related to distinct biological pathways. An increase in glycolysis was indicated by decreased abundance of glycogen and glucose and higher abundance of lactate. Several amino acids, as well as xanthine and other intermediates of nucleotide metabolism, such as inosine, uracil, uridine, and ATP, were found in higher concentrations in samples from infected animals. Finally, several compounds indicate a generalized oxidative stress during Mtb infection. Consistent with this finding, a signature of oxidative stress was revealed by metabolic profiling of granulomas in Mtb-infected guinea pigs.[42]

In a comparison of TB patients with LTBIs and uninfected healthy controls for abundance of 428 serum metabolites,[43] over 170 showed significant differences. The metabolites were clustered by correlation of their abundances to improve data integration. Clusters showing significant differences between the study groups included lysophosphatidylcholines, bile acids, uremic toxins, and amino acids. Two clusters were of particular interest. First, a signature of oxidative stress was linked to a cluster involving inosine degradation products (hypoxanthine, xanthine, and ribose), as well as to other molecules related to maintenance of the redox potential. Second, a smaller cluster comprising three forms of fibrinopeptide A indicated active processes underlying granuloma formation, notably walling off lesions from surrounding tissue. Furthermore, a decrease in tryptophan quantity and a reciprocal increase in that of kynurenine—a product of tryptophan degradation through IDO—were observed. However, the levels of these metabolites were not strongly correlated, suggesting that the decrease of tryptophan is most likely not due to IDO activity directly. Although this might be surprising at first sight, it is easily explained by the fact that (1) tryptophan is involved in several metabolic pathways, and (2) absolute plasma tryptophan levels exceed the abundance of kynurenines by at least an order of magnitude.[44] Intriguingly, the established biosignatures showed error rates in the range of 4–6%, with approximately the same number of false-positives and false-negatives, on par with the results from transcriptome analyses.

Challenges in high-throughput profiling

It is beyond doubt that HT platforms, such as transcriptomic and metabolic profiling, can provide deeper insight into infectious disease pathogenesis. For practical use, biosignatures need to include a limited number of variables, which must be analyzed in a cost-effective setting. For transcriptomics, universal readout systems exist, the most straightforward one being a custom-made PCR-based test. By contrast, a single readout platform does not exist for metabolomics. Moreover, quantities of metabolites are relative within a given experimental setup, and it is impossible to directly join or compare results from different studies.

In a diagnostic setting, samples from organs directly affected by the pathogen (e.g., lung tissue in TB) are generally not available. From the standpoint of point-of-care diagnosis, samples that can be easily collected in a field setting, such as urine or peripheral blood, would be preferable. Thus, a cost-effective test will need to target variables that reflect pathology at the local site of infection, imposing limits on the variables that can be analyzed. For example, transcriptomics catches the response of peripheral blood cells, and metabolic profiling allows better understanding of biological processes that result from host–pathogen interactions at the site of infection. Thus, different HT platforms have different strengths, which contribute to a more multifaceted biomarker profile. Taking advantage of this will be an important challenge for future biomarker research.

External validations and comparisons

A pathognomonic, clinically applicable biosignature of a disease needs to be both specific and sensitive. To date, many HT analyses have focused on a comparison between two groups (generally, disease vs. control), but even though a low error rate can be achieved in such a set up, it is insufficient from a translational point of view. While different diseases can trigger similar mechanisms, a biosignature appropriate for clinical diagnosis needs to be uniquely specific for the targeted disease. In the case of TB, HT studies have primarily focused on discrimination between active TB patients and healthy controls. Although these studies can unveil critical biological processes underlying TB, they are mostly indicative for a general pathological state of persistent immune activation.

A few studies, however, have attempted to compare biosignatures for TB with other diseases to unravel TB-specific biomarkers.[14,45–47] In comparing expression patterns of TB with those of other infectious diseases, Berry *et al.*[14] derived a distinct transcriptional signature comprising 86 genes. Subsequently, we showed that this signature is highly similar in patients with TB and pulmonary sarcoidosis (SARC),[45] another chronic inflammatory lung disease with similar pathologic appearance but distinct etiology. A similar overlap between TB and SARC was observed by Koth *et al.*[48] when comparing TB signatures from the study by Berry *et al.*[14] with their own gene expression profiles in SARC patients.

The clinical similarities between TB and SARC are reflected by highly matched expression signatures of both gene transcripts and microRNAs. This resemblance mirrors general immunopathological mechanisms underlying both diseases rather than disease-specific features. An earlier analysis revealed a high enrichment in TB of genes involved in systemic lupus erythematosus (SLE), further emphasizing similarities in gene expression signatures between the different disease entities.[14,15] Intriguingly, the characteristic markers distinguishing TB patients from healthy controls, including interferon and Fc gamma receptor signaling, complement activation, and TLR signaling, were shared by both diseases.

On the other hand, a sufficiently large number of markers unique for either TB or SARC were identified.[45] Gene expression profiles from TB patients indicated elevated metabolic activity compared to profiles from SARC patients. This included higher protein turnover and enrichment for genes involved in the electron transport chain. SARC patients presented a highly significant increase of matrix metallopeptidase 14 (MMP14) that was not observed in TB patients nor in healthy controls. Another significant difference between both diseases was the elevated expression of defense response genes in TB patients, mirroring the infectious nature of TB disease versus noninfectious SARC.[45]

Together, these results underscore the similarity of the immunopathologic processes operative in distinct diseases but also disease-specific mechanisms, thus calling for comparative validation studies in diverse cohorts and in comparison with different diseases. Elucidation of commonalities and singularities of distinct disease entities is not only critical to specificity but also to the understanding of mechanisms underlying pathogenicity. Groups of functions, processes, and pathways shared between several diseases can be treated as modules, from which both disease-specific profiles and clusters of diseases with similar underlying pathology can be constructed.

In addition, biology-directed evaluation of biomarker profiles can provide important insights. While it may be tempting to treat a particular HT data set as a kind of black box used for diagnostic purposes, focusing on summary statistics and low machine learning error rates, it can be equally rewarding to study functional implications of the results and consider their biological interpretations. HT methods, such as transcriptomic or metabolic profiling, are often hampered by the conundrum of multiple testing not the least because a large number of statistical tests can either cause a high false-positive ratio or, after inclusion of appropriate corrections for multiple testing, lead to lowered sensitivity. In contrast, in a hypothesis-generating framework, this is less of an issue, since false-positive statements can be tested *a posteriori* with more sensitive, low-throughput methods.

Future directions for high-throughput biomarker discovery

The potential of HT methods to define novel and composite biosignatures is beyond doubt. However, translation of a biosignature into a diagnostic measure requires validation of large sample sizes in large numbers of diverse cohorts, making HT methods not practicable and/or prohibitively expensive. In the case of RNA analyses, it is relatively straightforward to develop an intermediate multiplex PCR with a selected number of genes. Furthermore, such validation tests must provide standardized or absolute values that are comparable between different studies.

An important tool in the discovery of relevant pathways and systems are multivariate and clustering analyses in which within-group, between-sample variance is used to experimentally form functionally related or coregulated variables. Given the highly multidimensional nature of the HT data, this allows stepping beyond a case-by-case inspection of significant results. Most importantly, however, this allows prediction of novel functional relationships that would otherwise remain unexplored, for example, by analyzing the correlations between entities (genes, metabolites, etc.). The need to explore the variance between individuals instead of treating it as a source of error is often neglected, especially in areas other than transcription studies, where expression-based gene clustering has long since become an irreplaceable tool of functional analysis.

Focusing on more than one platform requires substantial efforts and resources. In the long term, robust biosignatures could emerge from combined sets of information stemming from different levels of regulation and different body compartments. A recently described multiplatform approach toward an enhanced perspective of the biological processes involved in pathogenesis employed proteome and transcriptome analyses to construct a robust sample classification.[49]

Concluding remarks and outlook

In conclusion, enormous efforts are still needed to solve some of the major challenges of unraveling biomarkers for TB.[50] We believe that an HT analysis of the host response in TB, which combines the strengths of different platforms, is best suited for a mechanistic interpretation of this disease. Ultimately, this will help to define biosignatures that diagnose different stages of TB, including risk of reactivation and progression to disease, as well as response to therapeutic and preventive measures.

It is increasingly accepted that biomarker research must include various aspects: state-of-the-art discovery techniques, solid clinical case definitions, careful epidemiologic characterization of study populations, and, last but not least, computational biology. A single biomarker will not suffice for TB diagnosis. Rather, a biosignature comprising a selected number of markers, which may stem from different analytical platforms, will likely be required. As a consequence, algorithms will need to be developed to distinguish not only health from disease, but also different types of disease and distinct stages of complex diseases. Sophisticated computational analyses will be required to ultimately define prognostic biosignatures that can predict risk of active TB in individuals with LTBI. Prognostic biosignatures would not only be of enormous value for identifying high-risk individuals, but also could facilitate preventive drug therapy. Moreover, they could reduce cost and duration of clinical trials by allowing stratification of high-risk individuals for inclusion in efficacy trials with novel drugs and vaccines. Clinical trial monitoring with biosignatures predicting the clinical endpoint would allow early decisions about efficacy of regimens under assessment, as in head-to-head vaccine trials to identify the most efficacious candidates or combinations thereof. At the same time, we wish to emphasize the importance of biomarker research for deeper insights into pathophysiological mechanisms underlying disease.

Biomarker research requires more intensive efforts and financial investment, in particular for validation across different cohorts, in diverse environmental settings, and in cases suffering from comorbidities. Yet, in the long run, a predictive biosignature will reduce cost by accelerating the transition of new products through the clinical trial pipeline and by improving TB diagnosis at the point of care. As an equally important result, biosignatures can create a basis for better understanding of the human host response (see Fig. 1). Countries in economic transition, such as India, are particularly relevant for such research directions since they combine high prevalences of TB with progress in biomedical research and development, providing unique opportunities for improved control measures for TB.

Acknowledgments

This work is supported by EU FP7 projects NEWT-BVAC (HEALTH-F3-2009-241745), TRANSVAC (FP7-INFRASTRUCTURES-2008-228403), and A-DITEC (HEALTH-F4-2011-280873) from the European Union; the European and Developing Countries Clinical Trials Partnership (EDCTP) project "Collaboration and integration of tuberculosis vaccine trials in Europe and Africa" (TBTEA, MS.20120.10800.002); the project "African European Tuberculosis Consortium" (AE-TBC); the Bill & Melinda Gates Foundation Grand Challenges in Global Health Program (BMGF GC6-74, #37772); and the Innovative Medicines Initiative Joint Undertaking "Biomarkers for Enhanced Vaccine Safety" BIOVACSAFE (IMI JU Grant No. 115308). The authors thank Mary Louise Grossman for help preparing the manuscript.

Conflicts of interest

S.H.E.K. is an advisor of Cellestis, Ltd.

References

1. World Health Organization. Global tuberculosis control 2011. 2011. World Health Organization. Geneva. Available at www.who.int/tb/publications/global_report/2011/en/index.html.
2. Kaufmann, S.H. 2011. Fact and fiction in tuberculosis vaccine research: 10 years later. *Lancet Infect. Dis.* **11:** 633–640.
3. Raviglione, M., B. Marais, K. Floyd, *et al.* 2012. Scaling up interventions to achieve global tuberculosis control: progress and new developments. *Lancet* **379:** 1902–1913.
4. Maertzdorf, J., I.J. Weiner & S.H. Kaufmann. 2012. Enabling biomarkers for tuberculosis control. *Int. J Tuberc. Lung Dis.* **16:** 1140–1148.
5. Boehme, C.C., M.P. Nicol, P. Nabeta, *et al.* 2011. Feasibility, diagnostic accuracy, and effectiveness of decentralised use of the Xpert MTB/RIF test for diagnosis of tuberculosis and multidrug resistance: a multicentre implementation study. *Lancet* **377:** 1495–1505.
6. Davies, P.D. & M. Pai. 2008. The diagnosis and misdiagnosis of tuberculosis. *Int. J. Tuberc. Lung Dis.* **12:** 1226–1234.
7. Philips, J.A. & J.D. Ernst. 2012. Tuberculosis pathogenesis and immunity. *Annu. Rev. Pathol.* **7:** 353–384.
8. Pai, M., K. Gokhale, R. Joshi, *et al.* 2005. Mycobacterium tuberculosis infection in health care workers in rural India: comparison of a whole-blood interferon gamma assay with tuberculin skin testing. *JAMA* **293:** 2746–2755.
9. Wallis, R.S., M. Pai, D. Menzies, *et al.* 2010. Biomarkers and diagnostics for tuberculosis: progress, needs, and translation into practice. *Lancet* **375:** 1920–1937.
10. Parida, S.K. & S.H. Kaufmann. 2010. The quest for biomarkers in tuberculosis. *Drug Discov. Today* **15:** 148–157.
11. Mistry, R., J.M. Cliff, C.L. Clayton, *et al.* 2007. Gene-expression patterns in whole blood identify subjects at risk for recurrent tuberculosis. *J. Infect. Dis.* **195:** 357–365.
12. Jacobsen, M., D. Repsilber, A. Gutschmidt, *et al.* 2007. Candidate biomarkers for discrimination between infection and disease caused by Mycobacterium tuberculosis. *J. Mol. Med.* **85:** 613–621.
13. Jacobsen, M., J. Mattow, D. Repsilber & S.H. Kaufmann. 2008. Novel strategies to identify biomarkers in tuberculosis. *Biol. Chem.* **389:** 487–495.
14. Berry, M.P., C.M. Graham, F.W. McNab, *et al.* 2010. An interferon-inducible neutrophil-driven blood transcriptional signature in human tuberculosis. *Nature* **466:** 973–977.
15. Maertzdorf, J., M. Ota, D. Repsilber, *et al.* 2011. Functional correlations of pathogenesis-driven gene expression signatures in tuberculosis. *PLoS One* **6:** e26938.
16. Maertzdorf, J., D. Repsilber, S.K. Parida, *et al.* 2011. Human gene expression profiles of susceptibility and resistance in tuberculosis. *Genes Immun.* **12:** 15–22.

17. Lesho, E., F.J. Forestiero, M.H. Hirata, *et al.* 2011. Transcriptional responses of host peripheral blood cells to tuberculosis infection. *Tuberculosis* **91:** 390–399.

18. Jacobsen, M., D. Repsilber, K. Kleinsteuber, *et al.* 2011. Suppressor of cytokine signaling-3 is affected in T-cells from tuberculosisTB patients. *Clin. Microbiol. Infect.* **17:** 1323–1331.

19. Walzl, G., K. Ronacher, W. Hanekom, *et al.* 2011. Immunological biomarkers of tuberculosis. *Nat. Rev. Immunol.* **11:** 343–354.

20. John, S.H., J. Kenneth & A.S. Gandhe. 2012. Host biomarkers of clinical relevance in tuberculosis: review of gene and protein expression studies. *Biomarkers* **17:** 1–8.

21. Djebali, S., C.A. Davis, A. Merkel, *et al.* 2012. Landscape of transcription in human cells. *Nature* **489:** 101–108.

22. O'Connell, R.M., D.S. Rao & D. Baltimore. 2012. microRNA regulation of inflammatory responses. *Annu. Rev. Immunol.* **30:** 295–312.

23. Moazed, D. 2009. Small RNAs in transcriptional gene silencing and genome defence. *Nature* **457:** 413–420.

24. Hassan, T., P.J. McKiernan, N.G. McElvaney, *et al.* 2012. Therapeutic modulation of miRNA for the treatment of proinflammatory lung diseases. *Expert Rev. Anti. Infect. Ther.* **10:** 359–368.

25. Wery, M., M. Kwapisz & A. Morillon. 2011. Noncoding RNAs in gene regulation. *Wiley Interdiscip. Rev. Syst. Biol. Med.* **3:** 728–738.

26. Wang, C., S. Yang, G. Sun, *et al.* 2011. Comparative miRNA expression profiles in individuals with latent and active tuberculosis. *PLoS One* **6:** e25832.

27. Fu, Y., Z. Yi, X. Wu, *et al.* 2011. Circulating microRNAs in patients with active pulmonary tuberculosis. *J. Clin. Microbiol.* **49:** 4246–4251.

28. Liu, Y., X. Wang, J. Jiang, *et al.* 2011. Modulation of T cell cytokine production by miR-144* with elevated expression in patients with pulmonary tuberculosis. *Mol. Immunol.* **48:** 1084–1090.

29. Wu, J., C. Lu, N. Diao, *et al.* 2012. Analysis of microRNA expression profiling identifies miR-155 and miR-155* as potential diagnostic markers for active tuberculosis: a preliminary study. *Hum. Immunol.* **73:** 31–37.

30. Dorhoi, A., M. Iannaccone, M. Farinacci, *et al.* The microRNA miR-223 constrains lethal inflammation during *Mycobacterium tuberculosis* infection. Submitted for publication.

31. Kaddurah-Daouk, R., B.S. Kristal & R.M. Weinshilboum. 2008. Metabolomics: a global biochemical approach to drug response and disease. *Annu. Rev. Pharmacol. Toxicol.* **48:** 653–683.

32. Griffin, J.L. & J.P. Shockcor. 2004. Metabolic profiles of cancer cells. *Nat. Rev. Cancer* **4:** 551–561.

33. Sabatine, M.S., E. Liu, D.A. Morrow, *et al.* 2005. Metabolomic identification of novel biomarkers of myocardial ischemia. *Circulation* **112:** 3868–3875.

34. Wang, T.J., M.G. Larson, R.S. Vasan, *et al.* 2011. Metabolite profiles and the risk of developing diabetes. *Nat. Med.* **17:** 448–453.

35. Jeon, C.Y. & M.B. Murray. 2008. Diabetes mellitus increases the risk of active tuberculosis: a systematic review of 13 observational studies. *PLoS Med.* **5:** e152.

36. Galon, J., D. Franchimont, N. Hiroi, *et al.* 2002. Gene profiling reveals unknown enhancing and suppressive actions of glucocorticoids on immune cells. *FASEB J.* **16:** 61–71.

37. Saric, J. 2010. Interactions between immunity and metabolism—contributions from the metabolic profiling of parasite-rodent models. *Parasitology* **137:** 1451–1466.

38. Hasko, G., D.G. Kuhel, Z.H. Nemeth, *et al.* 2000. Inosine inhibits inflammatory cytokine production by a posttranscriptional mechanism and protects against endotoxin-induced shock. *J. Immunol.* **164:** 1013–1019.

39. Slupsky, C.M., K.N. Rankin, H. Fu, *et al.* 2009. Pneumococcal pneumonia: potential for diagnosis through a urinary metabolic profile. *J. Proteome Res.* **8:** 5550–5558.

40. Laiakis, E.C., G.A. Morris, A.J. Fornace & S.R. Howie. 2010. Metabolomic analysis in severe childhood pneumonia in the Gambia, West Africa: findings from a pilot study. *PLoS One* **5**(9): pii: e12655.

41. Shin, J.H., J.Y. Yang, B.Y. Jeon, *et al.* 2011. H NMR-based metabolomic profiling in mice infected with Mycobacterium tuberculosis. *J. Proteome Res.* **10:** 2238–2247.

42. Somashekar, B.S., A.G. Amin, C.D. Rithner, *et al.* 2011. Metabolic profiling of lung granuloma in Mycobacterium tuberculosis infected guinea pigs: ex vivo 1H magic angle spinning NMR studies. *J. Proteome Res.* **10:** 4186–4195.

43. Weiner, J., III, S.K. Parida, J. Maertzdorf, *et al.* 2012. Biomarkers of inflammation, immunosuppression and stress with active disease are revealed by metabolomic profiling of tuberculosis patients. *PLoS One* **7:** e40221.

44. de Jong, W.H., R. Smit, S.J. Bakker, *et al.* 2009. Plasma tryptophan, kynurenine and 3-hydroxykynurenine measurement using automated on-line solid-phase extraction HPLC-tandem mass spectrometry. *J Chromatogr. B Analyt. Technol. Biomed. Life Sci.* **877:** 603–609.

45. Maertzdorf, J., J. Weiner, III, H.J. Mollenkopf, *et al.* 2012. Common patterns and disease-related signatures in tuberculosis and sarcoidosis. *Proc. Natl. Acad. Sci. USA* **109:** 7853–7858.

46. Phillips, M., V. Basa-Dalay, G. Bothamley, *et al.* 2010. Breath biomarkers of active pulmonary tuberculosis. *Tuberculosis* **90:** 145–151.

47. Sandhu, G., F. Battaglia, B.K. Ely, *et al.* 2012. Discriminating active from latent tuberculosis in patients presenting to community clinics. *PLoS One* **7:** e38080.

48. Koth, L.L., O.D. Solberg, J.C. Peng, *et al.* 2011. Sarcoidosis blood transcriptome reflects lung inflammation and overlaps with tuberculosis. *Am. J. Respir. Crit. Care Med.* **184:** 1153–1163.

49. Blanchet, L., A. Smolinska, A. Attali, *et al.* 2011. Fusion of metabolomics and proteomics data for biomarkers discovery: case study on the experimental autoimmune encephalomyelitis. *BMC. Bioinform.* **12:** 254.

50. Ottenhoff, T.H., J.J. Ellner & S.H. Kaufmann. 2012. Ten challenges for TB biomarkers. *Tuberculosis* **92**(Suppl 1): S17–S20.

Ann. N.Y. Acad. Sci. ISSN 0077-8923

ANNALS OF THE NEW YORK ACADEMY OF SCIENCES
Issue: *Translational Immunology in Asia-Oceania*

Clinical relevance of antibody development in renal transplantation

Narinder Mehra, Jamshaid Siddiqui, Ajay Baranwal, Sanjeev Goswami, and Gurvinder Kaur

Department of Transplant Immunology and Immunogenetics, All India Institute of Medical Sciences, New Delhi, India

Address for correspondence: Prof. Narinder Mehra, Head, Department of Transplant Immunology and Immunogenetics, All India Institute of Medical Sciences, Ansari Nagar, New Delhi-110029, India. narin98@hotmail.com

The detection and characterization of anti-HLA antibodies and the clinical impact of their appearance following renal transplantation are areas of immense interest. In particular, *de novo* development of donor-specific antibodies (DSA) has been associated with acute and chronic antibody-mediated graft rejection (AMR). Recently, methods for antibody detection have evolved remarkably from conventional cell-based assays to advanced solid phase systems. These systems have revolutionized the art of defining clinically relevant antibodies that are directed toward a renal graft. While anti-HLA DSAs have been widely associated with poor graft survival, the role of non-HLA antibodies, particularly those directed against endothelial cells, is beginning to be realized. Appreciation of the mechanisms underlying T cell recognition of alloantigens has generated great interest in the use of synthetic peptides to prevent graft rejection. Hopefully, continued progress in unraveling the molecular mechanisms of graft rejection and posttransplant monitoring of antibodies using highly sensitive testing systems will prove beneficial to immunological risk assessment and early prediction of renal allograft failure.

Keywords: renal transplantation; donor-specific antibodies; non-HLA antibodies; graft rejection

Introduction

Renal transplantation has come a long way since Murray and his team first successfully transplanted a human kidney between identical twins in 1954.[1] Impressive advancements have been witnessed not only in transplant technology, but also in understanding the immunological aspects, including developments in newer and more robust immunosuppressive protocols leading to steady improvement in graft outcomes. Currently, kidney transplantation has become the preferred choice for treating patients with end-stage renal disease, since it not only improves the quality of life as measured by added years, but also is cost-effective compared to hemodialysis. Nevertheless, despite such advances in immunological monitoring, chronic rejection remains a challenge, and long-term outcomes following renal transplantation still remain disappointing. While multiple factors have been shown to contribute to a progressive decline in allograft function and ultimate graft loss, increasing attention has been focused on the antibody-mediated component of allograft injury.

The human leukocyte antigen (HLA) system is a part of the major histocompatibility complex (MHC), which plays a critical role in regulating the immune response. The MHC molecules bind peptide fragments derived from protein antigens (e.g., viruses, bacterial peptides, and mismatched transplant antigens) and display them on the surface of professional antigen presenting cells (APCs), evoking effector responses upon recognition by T cell receptor. Four inherent features of the HLA system make it such an important immune response control system: extraordinary high polymorphism of its genes at the population level, tight linkage among its various loci, nonrandom association of its alleles, and its multipeptide binding ability. Developments in histocompatibility have largely been related to progress in technology, particularly computer aided programs of data storage and analysis. The major clinical role of HLA testing

doi: 10.1111/nyas.12034

 Ann. N.Y. Acad. Sci. 1283 (2013) 30–42 © 2013 New York Academy of Sciences.

remains in donor selection in organ and stem cell transplantation. In recent years, advancements in molecular HLA technologies have made the system an invaluable tool for population genetic studies and for defining susceptibility and/or protection genes in various disease conditions. The classical HLA genes are the most polymorphic in the human genome, with a large number of allelic variants at each locus.[2] Currently 8016 HLA alleles have become known (www.ebi.ac.uk/imgt/hla/). Data generated by most transplant centers have indicated an HLA matching effect with excellent graft outcome based on the degree of match grade, while poorly matched recipients are most likely to raise antibodies against the allograft.

Transplant recipients often produce anti-HLA antibodies as a result of previous exposure to allogeneic HLA molecules due to pregnancy, previous transplants, or blood transfusions from third party donors. Preformed anti-HLA antibodies in the recipient have been shown to cause hyperacute rejection of a donor kidney bearing the relevant HLA specificities. Therefore, detection of donor-specific anti-HLA antibodies (HLA DSA) before transplantation is an important step for assessing the patient's immunological risk and for excluding incompatible donors. Further, *de novo* development of HLA antibodies following transplantation has been repeatedly associated with allograft rejection, decreased allograft function, and even increased risk of renal allograft loss.[3–9] However, not all DSAs cause deterioration of the allograft function, rejection, or graft loss. The reasons for this are not completely understood; however, the ability to activate complement may be an important distinguishing factor differentiating pathogenic from nonpathogenic DSA.[10,11]

Although the critical role of antibodies in hyperacute rejection has been well known since the 1960s,[12] their significance in other forms of rejection was recognized only recently due to advances in more sensitive antibody detection technologies, such as of enzyme-linked immunosorbent assay (ELISA), flow cytometry, and multiplex quantitation assays such as Luminex®. While conventional flow cytometry crossmatch is among the most sensitive techniques permitting detection of all types of antibodies, including cell subset analysis, Luminex allows a more sensitive assessment of immunological risk at thresholds below those that can result in hyperacute rejection. These technologies have shifted the focus

from simply identifying patients at high risk of graft rejection to developing a gradient of immunological risk assessment for individual patients. Further, the recently introduced flow-based solid phase assay systems that use purified single antigen beads have provided an opportunity to detect HLA epitope-specific antibodies.[13]

Immunobiology of transplantation

The real first attempt to transplant a human kidney was made by the Ukranian surgeon Prof Yurii Voronoy in 1933, but this led to the disastrous consequence of immediate rejection of the organ and death of the patient. This was later attributed to blood group incompatibility between the recipient and donor. This rapid immune response is termed *hyperacute rejection* and is mediated by antibodies. Today kidney, pancreas, heart, lungs, liver, bone marrow, and cornea transplantations are routinely performed among unrelated individuals, with increasing frequency and with an impressive rate of success at least in the initial years following transplantation. Nevertheless long-term survival remains an area of concern. Despite dramatic short-term improvements in graft survival, there has been little significant change in long-term graft survival rates in the last two decades. For example, the half-life of survival of recipients who received transplants from deceased donors has increased gradually over a period of time from 6.6 years in 1989 and 8 years in 1995 to just about 8.8 years by 2005. Similarly, for recipients of transplants from living donors, half-life was 11.4 years in 1989 and 11.9 years in 2005.[14] Substantial numbers of grafts fail due to appearance of cytotoxic antibodies, the majority of which are HLA specific, though the role of non-HLA-specific antibodies is also beginning to be recognized.

Antigen processing and presentation

Professional APCs possess machinery to detect and degrade antigens into small peptides (processing), bind them to MHC molecules, and then express them as peptide/MHC complexes on their cell surfaces. Whether the processed antigen peptide links preferentially to class I or class II MHC molecules depends upon the way the antigen enters the cell. The endogeneous protein antigens in cytosol (cytoplasm) get bound to class I MHC for presentation to CD8+ cytotoxic T lymphocytes, while those in vesicles (exogeneous) get loaded onto class II MHC

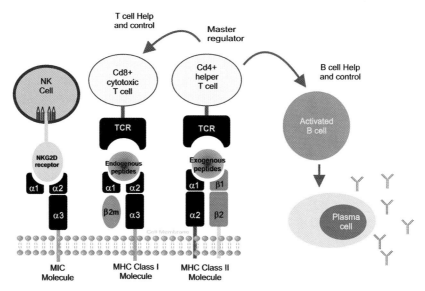

Figure 1. MHC class I and II molecules along with their bound peptides interact with the T cell receptor on the surface of CD8[+] and CD4[+] T cells presenting endogeneous and exogenously generated peptides, respectively. The CD4[+] helper T cells act as master regulators, helping and controlling the CD8[+] cytotoxic T cells, on one hand, and B cells on the other, leading to antibody formation by the plasma cells. The MHC class I chain–related gene A (MICA) is also a highly polymorphic molecule that engages the NKG2D receptor on the surface of natural killer (NK) cells. Unlike MHC classes I and II, this molecule does not have an associated light chain.

for inspection by the CD4[+] helper T cells. Within the APCs, endogeneous antigens (those that are produced within the cytoplasm) are tagged by ubiquitin and degraded by cytoplasmic proteasomes. The degraded peptides are then transported into the rough endoplasmic reticulum (RER) via transporters associated with antigen processing (TAP1 and TAP2). An antigen peptide then slips into the peptide binding groove of a class I molecule that has been synthesized in the rough endoplasmic reticulum. The MHC class I/antigen peptide complex is then transported through the Golgi complex to the cell surface of APCs for presentation to the CD8[+] cytotoxic T cells (Fig. 1).

MHC class II heterodimer, after synthesis in the RER, binds to invariant chain and this complex is then transported to late endosomes, where the invariant chain is degraded into a small fragment known as the class II invariant chain peptide (CLIP). The CLIP remains bound to the peptide binding groove of the class II molecule. Exogeneous antigens (those that are produced outside the cell), after being processed into antigenic peptides in the endosomal/lysosomal system of APCs, are exchanged with CLIP with the help of HLA-DM. The MHC class II/antigen peptide complex is then transported

to the cell surface of the APC for presentation to the CD4[+] T cells.

The third important molecule, the MHC class I chain–related gene A (MICA), is also polymorphic and engages the NKG2D receptor on the surface of natural killer (NK) cells.

Allorecognition

Allorecognition is defined as T cell recognition of MHC molecules between genetically disparate individuals of the same species. There are three different but not mutually exclusive pathways of allorecognition, namely direct, indirect, and the recently defined semidirect allorecognition. The direct pathway results when intact donor MHC molecules on the surface of donor antigen presenting cells (dAPCs), are presented to and recognized by recipient T cells. It is now recognized that this pathway predominates during the early posttransplant period and is the major factor mediating acute rejection. The dAPCs expressing donor alloantigens rapidly migrate from the graft and enter the secondary lymphoid tissues where they can encounter and prime allospecific T cells.[15] In the indirect pathway, on the other hand, donor histocompatibility molecules are internalized, processed and presented as peptides by recipient antigen presenting cells (rAPCs) to recipient T lymphocytes. In recent years, the indirect pathway has gained recognition because of its role in sustaining the ongoing, persistent response fueled by epitope spreading as a variety of allopeptides are successively presented by rAPCs. In general, the direct pathway plays a dominant role in acute rejection while the indirect pathway is associated with chronic rejection, as is evident both in the animal model systems as well as clinical settings.[16,17] The endothelial cells derived from recipients may also play a role in the indirect allorecognition pathway.[18,19] The endothelium of allograft can be replaced by recipient cells that in turn can present alloantigens to host immune cells via the indirect pathway. In the semidirect pathway of allorecognition, the host T cells interact with rAPCs that have acquired intact donor MHC: peptide complexes from donor cells. The exact mechanism of semidirect allorecognition in transplant rejection and tolerance is not fully clear.

In the classical immune pathway, CD4[+] T cell acts as the "headquarters cell" that helps and supports the CD8[+] effector T cells on one hand and B cells on the other. Transplants carried out between HLA mismatched donor–recipient pairs have the greater chance of rejection due to development of donor-specific antibodies compared to those between better matched grafts. Data collated at the CTS registry have indicated that over a period of time the impact of HLA matching becomes distinctively evident, due to deteriorating graft survival rates in poorly matched grafts. The data provide evidence to suggest that the better the match grade between the recipient and the donor, the lesser the chances of antibody development and subsequent rejection.[20]

Antibody-mediated rejection

The past decade has witnessed three very important developments that have influenced our understanding of antibody-mediated rejection (AMR): (1) the discovery of the detrimental effect of donor-specific anti-HLA antibodies on allograft survival and their association with AMR, (2) the advent of newer and more sensitive techniques for detection of DSA, and (3) revisions in Banff criteria for assessment of graft pathology. The main mechanisms implicated in immunological events leading to graft deterioration include cell-mediated cytotoxicity, delayed type hypersensitivity, and antibody-dependent cellular cy-

totoxicity.[21] Direct antibody mediated damage due to the development of donor-specific alloantibody induced rejection supports the importance of antibodies in graft rejection.[22] Several investigators have reported that the pre and posttransplant development of IgG donor-directed antibodies predict the risk of both acute and chronic allograft rejection.[5,23–25]

Alloantibodies preferentially attack peritubular and glomerular capillaries of the transplanted kidney. The target antigens in AMR are most often situated on the endothelium, resulting in the histopathological findings of acute (glomerulitis, peritubular capillaritis) and chronic (transplant glomerulopathy) vascular injury. Endothelial damage also results in platelet activation and microthrombus formation. Of critical importance is C4d deposition, which is regarded as an important surrogate marker for the diagnosis of hyperacute and acute humoral rejection.[26,27] Recent reports have provided a convincing proof that C4d deposition is strongly associated with the development of HLA class I and II antibodies directed against donor antigens.[28–30] Presently this is the most widely accepted marker of complement fixing circulating antibodies to the endothelium.

Antibody detection techniques

The two main goals associated with organ transplantation are increased access to transplantation for better quality of life and improved graft outcome to significantly increase the duration that the grafted organ can remain in the new host. The most important factor in organ transplantation is the meticulous evaluation of the possible occurrence of antidonor antibodies before transplantation. Since antibodies cause graft rejection, technologies for their detection must be sufficiently sensitive to predict hyperacute or humoral rejection and adequately specific to determine immunological failure. An optimal combination of the two elements is necessary to determine the predictive value of individual techniques. Currently, anti-HLA antibodies can be detected by a number of techniques that include target donor cell-based crossmatch assays, such as complement-dependent cytotoxicity (CDC) and flow cytometry crossmatch (FCXM), and HLA protein–based (solid phase) assays, such as an enzyme-linked immunoabsorbent assay (ELISA) or HLA antigen-coated fluorescence bead assay

Table 1. A summary of the various methodologies used for antibody detection for renal transplant purposes[31–39,45,46]

	CDC	ELISA	FCXM	SPA (Luminex)
Sensitivity	+	++	+++	++++
Specificity	+++	+	++	+++
HLA antibodies	+	+	+	+
Non-HLA antibodies	+	−	+	+ (MICA)
C-fixing antibodies	+	+	+	+
Non-C fixing	−	+	+	+
Subclass	IgG1, G3, IgM	IgG1, G2, G3, G4	IgG1, G2, G3, G4, IgA, IgM	IgG1, G2, G3, G4
Live cell requirement	+	−	+	−
Advantages	Functional assay	Detects both C and non-C fixing antibodies	Detects all antibodies, cell subset analyses (important in sensitized/retransplant patients)	Identifies donor-specific antibodies (virtual crossmatch)
Limitations	Misses non-C-fixing antibodies, low antigen expression	Misses non HLA antibodies	False +/− results	False +/− results—no consensus on optimal MFI values

ABBREVIATIONS: CDC, complement-dependent cytotoxicity; FCXM, flow cytometry crossmatch; SPA, solid phase assay; MFI, mean fluorescence intensity

systems. Table 1 summarizes the available techniques for detection of anti-HLA and donor-specific antibodies along with their specific features and limitations.

Complement-dependent cytotoxicity assay. Introduced in the 1960s, the CDC crossmatch assay remains an essential requirement before transplantation.[12,31] In this assay, target lymphocytes are killed by antibody-activated complement when the recipient has preexisting antibodies or those developed *de novo* following transplantation. The main advantage of this assay is that it specifically detects antibodies that are capable of activating the complement. It is the only assay with a functional readout that may mimic the *in vivo* reality. The greatest drawback of the CDC assay is that it often misses low titer antibodies, resulting in false negatives, or gives rise to false positive results due to the detection of non-HLA antibodies and autoantibodies or high background reading due to spontaneous cell death (especially B cells). In addition, the assay is relatively time consuming, requires the isolation of T and/or B lymphocyte subpopulations from donor periph-

eral blood, and detects only complement fixing antibodies (IgG and IgM). Further, the test results are dependent largely on the level of cell surface antigen expression and the assay is less sensitive in detecting antidonor antibodies than the flow cytometry–based crossmatch.[32,33]

Flow cytometry crossmatch. The flow crossmatch technique was developed primarily to address some of the problems inherent to the CDC assay. Since the test can detect both complement fixing (IgG and IgM) and nonfixing (e.g., IgA) antibodies, it readily gained greater acceptance. It is a less subjective, quantitative method with 10- to 250-fold greater sensitivity than the CDC test and it is able to detect both low titre circulating alloantibodies and those directed against HLA class I (T cell FCXM) or class II (B cell FCXM) determinants. Further, FCXM does not require physically isolating lymphocyte subpopulations. In contrast to the traditional CDC test, FCXM is not a functional test because it only provides information on the binding of the donor-specific antibody to its potential donor target (expressed as channel shift) and not on the killing of the target. Accordingly, a positive FCXM (channel shift >50) does not necessarily mean that the bound antibodies have any pathological effect on the target cells. Antibody detection by flow cytometry does not reflect the ability of that antibody to activate complement: this is the major disadvantage of this technique.

Purified HLA antigen–based enzyme-linked immunoabsorbent assay (HLA-Ag ELISA). An ELISA-based HLA antibody detection method was commercially developed in the mid 1990s[34] as a more sensitive and less time-consuming technique for detecting primarily anti-HLA antibodies. A panel of mixture containing class I and/or class II HLA antigens, purified from culture supernatants or cell lysates from Epstein–Barr virus transformed lymphoblastoid cell lines, is coated on to the ELISA plates. After incubation of the coated plates with the test serum, the bound antibodies are detected using a peroxidase conjugated antihuman immunoglobulin antibody. Absorbance is read using an ELISA reader and the assay results analyzed using software. Recently, single HLA class I and class II antigens, instead of purified antigen mixture, have been tried as coating antigens. This purified HLA antigen–based ELISA test is highly sensitive, comparable to flow cytometry or the recently adopted Luminex-based assay system. It has been argued that the high sensitivity of this assay might be due to the greater amount of HLA antigens used to coat the ELISA plate. The viability of this assay as a clear indicator of the amount of antibody detected is questionable, since the test uses quantities of HLA antigens much greater than the normal biologic expression on the immune cell.

Luminex technology. This latest acquired technology has completely transformed the histocompatibility laboratory's approach and ability to detect HLA antibodies. Current data indicate that the Luminex platform is one of the most sensitive of the solid-phase antibody detection techniques that enable identification of antibody specificities in highly reactive sera.[35,36] The technique has been successfully applied to monitor patient antibody profiles in relation to particular specificities, such as following antibody removal strategies at pretransplant stage, and for identification of donor-specific antibodies posttransplantation. The biggest advantage of this technique is the single antigen bead system

that permits detection of epitope-specific antibodies to individual and specific HLA alleles and thus provides information on the virtual crossmatch.[37] The mean fluorescence intensity (MFI) of the beads is a measure of the amount and strength of the antibody present. Most centers concur that peak MFI >6000 is associated with poor graft outcomes,[38] although controversy exists on the optimum MFI cutoffs for classifying the antibody as positive or negative, particularly if it is HLA-DSA. Most centers agree that HLA-DSA with MFI >2000 should be considered clinically significant.[39] In our center, MFI >1000 is not ignored, because it indicates possible positivity of donor-specific antibodies, which can lead to accelerated acute rejection in a proportion of patients. Others have also suggested that an MFI cutoff value of 1000 for DSA provides a more valuable result in the context of clinical correlation.[40] Further, peak MFI in the recipient serum is considered a better indicator of graft survival than the MFI in the current sera, particularly if it is HLA-DSA.

Being highly sensitive, the Luminex technology often provides false positive results, leading to unnecessary delays on the waiting list. The biggest limitation of the technology is that it does not discriminate between complement fixing and non-complement fixing antibodies. This is important in the light of recent observations suggesting that noncomplement fixing antibodies (IgG2 and IgG4) could be as deleterious to the graft as the complement fixing ones (IgG1 and IgG3).[41] Further, the current panel of single HLA flow beads do not cover the whole diversity of HLA alleles. Hence populations like the Asian Indian that are characterized by a large number of novel alleles and unique HLA haplotypes[42,43] will be at a disadvantage because antibodies raised against such HLA alleles are likely to be missed. Current protocols rely primarily on defining antibodies directed against broad HLA specificities (e.g., HLA-DRB1*04, *15) without taking into consideration the allelic subtypes at four point difference (e.g., DRB1*0401 versus *0404). Since the allelic subtypes vary among and between different ethnic groups, the possibility of antibody development in relation to subtype difference between the donor and the recipient needs to be evaluated. Accordingly, improvements in Luminex-based antibody detection methods will become necessary. Another limitation of this technology is that not all HLA antibodies detected by single flow beads may

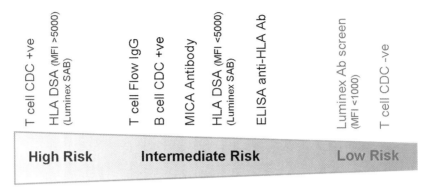

Figure 2. Pretransplant donor–recipient work-up in relation to antibody detection. Patients with a CDC IgG crossmatch positive for T cells and evidence of high titer donor-specific antibodies (DSA) detected by Luminex single antigen beads (SAB) are at highest risk.

in fact be clinically relevant. The assay may also provide false positive results and the detected HLA antibodies may only be of limited clinical relevance even in the presence of a true positive result. Luminex beads accommodate both intact as well as denatured HLA molecules. The natural HLA antibodies present in nonimmunized individuals react preferentially with these denatured molecules. A recent study has shown that antibodies reactive to these denatured HLA molecules are clinically irrelevant.[44] Further, binding of the solubilized class I molecules on beads may alter the tertiary structure of the antigen leading to false negative and/or positive reactions when human monoclonal antibodies directed against class I molecules are used as detecting reagents.[45] Similar reactions may occur with sera from potential transplant recipients.[46]

Anti-HLA antibodies: pretransplantation level
There is universal agreement that pretransplant HLA class I and class II antibodies individually or in combination are associated with poor allograft outcome following renal transplantation.[38,47–49] Detection of these antibodies has become more precise and specific with the use of the Luminex single antigen bead assay system. However, the exact clinical significance of antibodies defined by this assay in the absence of a positive CDC crossmatch requires further evaluation. Based on current experience, an assessment of the gradient of risk prediction can be of immense value in helping the transplant team to plan a pretransplant work-up. Studies done by us[50] and others[51] have shown that patients who develop both anti-HLA class I and II antibodies experienced more frequent rejection episodes than those having

either of these antibodies alone. The latter study has also highlighted the importance of A, B, and DR mismatches in the presence of HLA class I and II antibodies. It has also been reported that the presence of class I and class II IgG DSA, as detected by single antigen bead in the pretransplant sera of renal recipients, is indicative of an increased risk for graft failure.[48]

Donor-specific HLA-DQ and DP antibodies are detectable only by the Luminex and flow cytometry assays, and they generally represent a low to intermediate level of immunological risk. However, if such antibodies give rise to an IgG positive B cell CDC crossmatch test, the level of immunological risk rises to intermediate or even high.[52] HLA-DP specific alloantibodies have traditionally been granted minimal significance because of the relatively low expression of DP antigens on renal endothelial cells. However, recent studies have suggested that donor-specific HLA-DP antibodies can mediate both acute and chronic allograft rejection just the same way as the anti-DR antibodies can.[53–56] A recent study by Gilbert *et al.*[57] has demonstrated the influence of pretransplant donor-specific HLA-C and DP antibodies on the development of acute humoral rejection episodes, that lead, in most cases, to graft failure. The study also revealed that anti-DP antibodies exerted more deleterious effect on graft outcome than anti-C antibodies.

Since the presence of antibodies is a major deterrent to the selection of a potential donor, an assessment of risk for graft rejection could provide a guide to donor selection (Fig. 2). It is important to know the level of antibodies as detected by more sensitive assays in the patient serum, since the low levels of pretransplant donor-specific antibodies are frequently clinically irrelevant.[39] Similarly, detection by highly sensitive methods should be critically analyzed before making a clinical decision.

Anti-HLA and donor-specific antibodies: de novo development

The impact of *de novo* development of class I and/or class II anti-HLA antibodies on acute or chronic allograft rejection is a subject of intense investigation. The development of such antibodies varies among individual patients. There is a lack of consensus on the time of onset of these antibodies, their intensity, duration, and associated graft dysfunction. It has been shown that *de novo* HLA class II DSA have greater influence on the development of antibody mediated injury and allograft failure than those against HLA class I alleles.[8,58] Alloantibodies formed within the first year of transplantation are much more damaging than those formed after completion of one year of transplantation.[59] Recently, the role of anti-DQ donor-specific antibodies has been highlighted with inferior renal allograft outcome.[60] This is an important observation since HLA-DQ expression is known to be upregulated in endothelial cells following renal transplantation[61] and may thus be an effective target for HLA-DQ antibodies. These results have highlighted the clinical importance of HLA-DQ (in addition to HLA-DR) matching in renal transplantation to define the risk associated with the development of DQ donor-specific antibodies.

It has been demonstrated that *de novo* development of nondonor-specific HLA antibodies is also associated with poor graft survival.[62–64] The presence of circulating anti-HLA antibodies and positive C4d stating on allograft biopsies correlate strongly with the development of acute and chronic rejection in kidney transplant recipients.[28,29] Hence, the very strong association between *de novo* production of donor-specific HLA antibodies and allograft failure highlights the importance of monitoring for posttransplant HLA antibodies as predictive biomarkers for allograft function. The clinical significance of IgM type anti-HLA antibodies in relation to allograft rejection is not clear. Studies using CDC and flow cytometry methods have suggested that IgM antibodies are generally not detrimental to the graft.[65] Others, however, have shown that a positive T cell IgM flow cytometry crossmatch at the time of transplant could be a risk factor for allograft rejection.[66]

C1q fixing antibodies. C1q is the first component of the classical complement pathway. Activation of the pathway begins with binding of an antibody to C1q. Once activated, the classical pathway leads to the formation of membrane attack complex, resulting in cell lysis and cell death. It is now recognized that not all DSAs lead to the development of AMR. In this respect, recent data have suggested that only those DSAs that are able to activate C1q are associated with a higher risk of AMR, compared to the C1q negative group.[48,67,68] In fact, only 47% of HLA-Ab specificities identified by Luminex–IgG could bind C1q, suggesting that about half of the IgG antibodies may not have an immediate or even late adverse effect on the graft.[69] In this complex and ever evolving field, one can conclude that complement mediated injury initiated by DSAs is responsible for most early AMR episodes. These studies have opened up novel therapeutic approaches toward preventing AMR by reducing deleterious donor-specific antibodies through inhibition of complement activation.

Non-HLA antibodies

In recent years, the focus has also shifted to the role of antibodies in renal transplantation other than those against HLA. Such non-HLA antibodies may also be clinically important in the development of allograft rejection, although the extent of their harmful effects is not fully clear.

Antiendothelial cell antibodies. Endothelial cells are critical to transplant outcomes in that they provide the initial contact point between the recipient's immune system and the transplanted allograft. Over the years, greater recognition of the role of antiendothelial cell antibodies (AECAs) in renal transplantation has provided researchers with an additional parameter to account for unexplained allograft losses. Several investigators have reported a significant correlation between the development of AECAs and hyperacute, accelerated, and acute renal rejections, even in situations involving HLA-identical sibling transplants.[70–75] The potential antigenic targets of AECAs that have been implicated with renal allograft rejection include angiotensin II type 1 receptor, vimentin, agrin (glomerular basement protein), and MICA.[76–79]

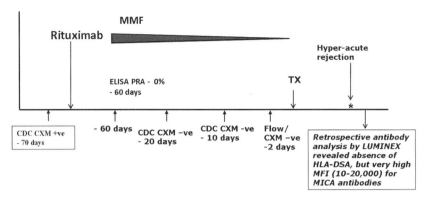

Figure 3. Time scale representation of antibody analysis in patient SS. The hyperacute rejection was linked to the presence of anti-MICA antibodies in the absence of HLA-DSA in the pretransplant serum. CDC, complement-dependent cytotoxicity; CXM, crossmatch.

Jackson *et al.*[80] conducted a study to assess the clinical relevance of donor-specific AECAs using donor-derived endothelial precursors. The study revealed a significantly higher incidence of allograft rejection in patients with donor reactive IgG AECAs. On further subtyping, these IgG antibodies were found to be mainly the IgG2 and IgG4 subclasses that do not activate complement. It was concluded that AECAs exert their action through endothelial cell activation, proliferation or apoptosis.

Major histocompatibility complex class I–related chain A. MICA is a highly polymorphic gene complex located within the MHC class I region of chromosome six and is known to have at least 84 alleles. It is constitutively expressed in endothelial cells, gut epithelial cells, skin-derived fibroblasts, monocytes, and keratinocytes, but not in immunocompetent cells.[81] An association between MICA antibodies and poor graft outcome in renal transplant recipients has been recognized in several studies.[8,82,83] Pretransplant MICA antibodies in kidney recipients were found to decrease graft survival, even when the recipients were well matched for HLA antigens and did not express HLA-specific antibodies.[84] We had reported earlier that the presence of both HLA-DSA and antidonor MICA antibodies in the recipient is a potentially disastrous combination, associated with very poor graft outcomes and even leading to hyperacute rejection in some cases.[50] The exact mechanism by which individuals develop antibodies against MICA is not clear. Both MICA and MICB (MHC class I chain–related gene B) are highly polymorphic antigenic molecules present on

endothelial cells and are therefore easy targets for humoral immunity associated with irreversible rejection of kidney allografts. It has been suggested that although pregnancy can induce the formation of such antibodies,[85] a role for blood transfusions is debatable.[84,86]

We present here the case report of a 15-year-old female, "SS," with end-stage renal disease and on maintenance hemodialysis, who was clinically and immunologically evaluated for renal transplantation. The patient with blood group A+ received a haploidentical kidney graft from her mother. The pretransplant CDC crossmatch was positive and the patient's panel reactive antibody test showed the presence of antibodies as defined by CDC- and ELISA-based tests (Fig. 3). The patient was treated with Rituximab and Mycophenolate mofetil (MMF) for eight weeks to remove any possible donor-specific antibodies, after which the CDC and flow cytometry crossmatch showed negative results. The renal transplantation was carried out but the patient underwent unexplained hyperacute rejection. A retrospective antibody evaluation by a single antigen bead-based Luminex assay revealed an absence of donor-specific HLA antibodies in the patient serum. However, the analysis of both pre and post-transplant serum samples showed the presence of MICA antibodies with MFI in the range 10,000–20,000. On stringent analysis it was concluded that the donor directed MICA antibody was the major risk factor for hyperacute rejection. The case highlights the need for including regular MICA antibody screening in the pretransplant work-up. Similar results have been published by other investigators, highlighting the role of pretransplant donor-specific MICA antibodies on the development of acute rejection.[87,88]

Antibody removal therapy

Current strategies used for prevention and treatment of antibody-mediated graft damage include (1) antibody removal and neutralization through plasmapheresis, immunoadsorption, intravenous immunoglobulin (IVIG) infusion, and splenectomy, (2) inhibition of B cell proliferation by using potent immunomodulatory agents that include Mycophenolate mofetil, rituximab, IVIG, and splenectomy, (3) proteasome-based plasma cell inhibitors like bortezomib, (4) T cell depleting agents that include antithymocyte globulin (ATG), (5) conversion to tacrolimus-based regimens, and (6) inhibition of complement pathway, for example, through blockage of the C5 component use of eculizumab. Of these, IVIG is the most commonly used strategy either alone or in combination with plasmapheresis. Indeed, IVIG at high dose without plasmapheresis has been performed successfully in pretransplant desensitization protocols and in the treatment of antibody-mediated rejection. Similarly, monoclonal antibody–based therapies have been successfully administered in the treatment of antibody-mediated graft rejection. These include anti-CD20 (rituximab)[89,90] and eculizumab, a humanized monoclonal antibody directed against the C5 component of complement, and other combination therapies. Use of these drugs has resulted in decreased plasmapheresis sessions. Further, bortezomib, a novel proteasome inhibitor, shows promise in the treatment of antibody mediated rejection.[91,92] Although, splenectomy has been successful in resistant AMR cases, the procedure has not gained importance because of the long-term possibilities of infections in immunocompromized individuals and the associated surgical risks.

Perspectives

The introduction of C4d staining in renal allograft biopsies and the advancement of more sensitive and specific techniques to detect antibodies have revolutionized our understanding about their role in determining risk stratification and treatment of antibody-mediated rejection. Substantial data demonstrate the association of *de novo* development of anti-HLA donor-specific and non-HLA antibodies with acute and chronic graft failure. However, further studies are needed to allow the community to reach a consensus on MFI cutoff values for the identification of harmful versus benign antibodies for accurate assessment of patients at increased risk of rejection. Bioinformatic tools like the HLA Matchmaker program[93] have been extremely valuable in defining cutoff MFI values for finding antibody reactivity for mismatched epitopes in sensitized patients. It is also important to define the effect of early versus late development of antibodies on allograft pathology for developing protocols for their neutralization. This, along with a clear understanding of the molecular mechanisms underlying graft rejection, will facilitate further refinements in immunosuppressive protocols and help to achieve the ultimate goal of long-term acceptance of the organ allograft through tolerance induction.

Acknowledgments

The authors thank the Department of Biotechnology (DBT), Ministry of Science and Technology, Government of India, and the Indian Council of Medical Research (ICMR) for financial assistance.

Conflicts of interest

The authors declare no conflicts of interest.

References

1. Murray, J.E., J.P. Merrill & J.H. Harrison. 1955. Renal homotransplantation between identical twins. *Surgical Forum* **6:** 432.

2. Mehra, N.K., G. Kaur, J. McCluskey, *et al.* 2010. *The HLA Complex in Biology and Medicine: A Resource Book.* Jaypee Brothers Medical Publishers (P) Ltd. New Delhi.

3. Halloran, P.F., J. Schlaut, K. Solez & N.S. Srinivasa. 1992. The significance of the anti-class I response: II. Clinical and pathologic features of renal transplants with anti-class I-like antibody. *Transplantation* **53:** 550–555.

4. Suthanthiran, M. & T.B. Strom. 1994. Medical progress: renal transplantation. *N. Engl. J. Med.* **331:** 365–376.

5. Terasaki, P. 2003. Humoral theory of transplantation. *Am. J. Transplant.* **3:** 665–673.

6. Hourmant, M., A. Cesbron-Gautier, P.I. Terasaki, *et al.* 2005. Frequency and clinical implications of development of donor specific and non-donor-specific HLA antibodies after kidney transplantation. *J. Am. Soc. Nephrol.* **16:** 2804–2812.

7. Terasaki, P. & M. Ozawa. 2005. Predictive value of HLA antibodies and serum creatinine in chronic rejection: results of a 2-year prospective trial. *Transplantation* **80:** 1194–1197.

8. Terasaki, P.I., M. Ozawa & R. Castro. 2007. Four-year follow-up of a prospective trial of HLA and MICA antibodies on kidney graft survival. *Am. J. Transplant.* **7:** 408–415.

9. Seveso, M., E. Bosio, E. Ancona & E. Cozzi. 2009. De novo anti-HLA antibody responses after renal transplantation: detection and clinical impact. *Contrib. Nephrol.* **162:** 87–98.

10. Wahrmann, M., M. Exner, M. Schillinger, *et al.* 2006. Pivotal role of complement-fixing HLA alloantibodies in presensitized kidney allograft recipients. *Am. J. Transplant.* **6:** 1033–1041.

11. Wahrmann, M., G. Bartel, M. Exner, *et al.* 2009. Clinical relevance of preformed C4d-fixing and non-C4d-fixing HLA single antigen reactivity in renal allograft recipients. *Transpl. Int.* **22:** 982–989.

12. Patel, R. & P.I. Terasaki. 1969. Significance of the positive crossmatch test in kidney transplantation. *N. Engl. J. Med.* **280:** 735–739.

13. Puttarajappa, C., R. Shapiro & H.P. Tan. 2012. Antibody mediated rejection in kidney transplantation: A review. *J. transplant.* **2012:** 1–9.

14. Lamb, K.E., S. Lodhi & H.U. Meier-Kriesche. 2011. Long-term renal allograft survival in the United States: a critical reappraisal. *Am. J. Transplant* **11:** 450–462.

15. Benichou, G. 1999. Direct and indirect antigen recognition: the pathways to allograft immune rejection. *Front. Biosci.* **4:** D476–D480.

16. Noorchashm, H., A.J. Reed, S.Y. Rostami, *et al.* 2006. B cell-mediated antigen presentation is required for the pathogenesis of acute cardiac allograft rejection. *J. Immunol.* **177:** 7715–7722.

17. Taylor, A.L., S.L. Negus, M. Negus, *et al.* 2007. Pathways of helper CD4 T cell allorecognition in generating alloantibody and CD8 T cell alloimmunity. *Transplantation* **83:** 931–937.

18. Grimm, P.C., P. Nickerson, J. Jeffery, *et al.* 2001. Neointimal and tubulointerstitial infiltration by recipient mesenchymal cells in chronic renal-allograft rejection. *N. Engl. J. Med.* **345:** 93–97.

19. Kapessidou, Y., C. Habran, S. Buonocore, *et al.* 2006. The replacement of graft endothelium by recipient-type cells conditions allograft rejection mediated by indirect pathway CD4+ T cells. *Transplantation* **82:** 582–591.

20. Opelz, G. & B. Dohler. 2007. Effect of human leukocyte antigen compatibility on kidney graft survival: comparative analysis of two decades. *Transplantation* **27:** 137–143.

21. Mason, D.W. & P.J. Morris. 1986. Effector mechanisms in allograft rejection. *Annu. Rev. Immunol.* **4:** 119–145.

22. Racusen, L.C., R.B. Colvin, K. Solez, *et al.* 2003. Antibody-mediated rejection criteria—an addition to the Banff 97 classification of renal allograft rejection. *Am. J. Transplant.* **3:** 708–714.

23. Francesca C., M. Pascual, N. Tolkoff-Rubin, *et al.* 2005. Prevalence and significance of anti-HLA and donor-specific antibodies long-term after renal transplantation. *Transpl. Int.* **18:** 532–540.

24. Terasaki, P.I. & J. Cai. 2005. Humoral theory of transplantation: further evidence. *Curr. Opin. Immunol.* **17:** 541–545.

25. Terasaki, P. & K. Mizutani. 2006. Antibody mediated rejection: update 2006. *Clin. J. Am. Soc. Nephrol.* **1:** 400–403.

26. Collins, A.B., E.E. Schneeberger, M.A. Pascual, *et al.* 1999. Complement activation in acute humoral renal allograft rejection: diagnostic significance of C4d deposits in peritubular capillaries. *J. Am. Soc. Nephrol.* **10:** 2208–2214.

27. Feucht, H.E., H. Schneeberger, G. Hillebrand, *et al.* 1993. Capillary deposition of C4d complement fragment and early renal graft loss. *Kidney Int.* **43:** 1333–1338.

28. Mauiyyedi, S., M. Crespo, A.B. Collins, *et al.* 2002. Acute humoral rejection in kidney transplantation II. Morphology, immunopathology, and pathologic classification. *J. Am. Soc. Nephrol.* **13:** 779–787.

29. Bohmig, G.A., M. Exner, A. Habicht, *et al.* 2002. Capillary C4d deposition in kidney allografts: a specific marker of alloantibody-dependent graft injury. *J. Am. Soc. Nephrol.* **13:** 1091–1099.

30. Haas, M., M.H. Rahman, L.C. Racusen, *et al.* 2006. C4d and C3d staining in biopsies of ABO- and HLA-incompatible renal allografts: correlation with histologic findings. *Am. J. Transplant.* **6:** 1829–1840.

31. Terasaki, P.I., T.L. Marchioro & T.E. Starzl. 1965. Sero-typing of human lymphocyte antigens: preliminary trials on long-term kidney homograft survivors. In *Histocompatibility Testing*: 83–96. National Academy of Sciences. National Research Council, Washington, DC.

32. Cook, D.J., P.I. Terasaki, Y. Iwaki, *et al.* 1987. An approach to reducing early kidney transplant failure by flow cytometry crossmatching. *Clin. Transplant.* **1:** 253–256.

33. Talbot, D. 1994. Flow cytometric crossmatching in human organ transplantation. *Transpl. Immunol.* **2:** 138–139.

34. Kao, K.J., J.C. Scornik & S.J. Small. 1993. Enzyme-linked immunoassay for anti-HLA antibodies—an alternative to panel studies by lymphocytotoxicity. *Transplantation* **55:** 192–196.

35. Gibney, E.M., L.R. Cagle, B. Freed, *et al.* 2006. Detection of donor specific antibodies using HLA coated microspheres: another tool for kidney transplant risk stratification. *Nephrol. Dial. Transplant.* **21:** 2625–2629.

36. Vaidya, S., D. Partlow, B. Susskind, *et al.* 2006. Prediction of crossmatch outcome of highly sensitised patients by single and/or multiple antigen bead luminex assay. *Transplantation* **82:** 1524–1528.

37. El-Awar, N., J.H. Lee, C. Tarsitani & P.I. Terasaki. 2007. HLA class I epitopes: recognition of binding sites by mAbs or eluted alloantibody confirmed with single recombinant antigens. *Hum. Immunol.* **68:** 170–180.

38. Lefaucheur, C., A. Loupy, G.S. Hill, *et al.* 2010. Preexisting donor-specific HLA antibodies predict outcome in kidney transplantation. *J. Am. Soc. Nephrol.* **21:** 1398–1406.

39. Aubert, V., J.P. Venetz, G. Pantaleo & M. Pascual. 2009. Low levels of human leukocyte antigen donor-specific antibodies detected by solid phase assay before transplantation are frequently clinically relevant. *Hum. Immunol.* **70:** 580–583.

40. Thammanichanond, D., A. Ingsathit, T. Mongkolsuk, *et al.* 2012. Pre-transplant donor specific antibody and its clinical significance in kidney transplantation. *Asian Pac. J. Allergy Immunol.* **30:** 48–54.

41. Honger, G., H. Hopfer, M.L. Arnold, *et al.* 2011. Pretransplant IgG subclasses of donor-specific human leukocyte antigen antibodies and development of antibody-mediated rejection. *Transplantation* **92:** 41–47.

42. Jaini, R., G. Kaur & N.K. Mehra. 2002. Heterogeneity of HLA-DRB1*04 and its associated haplotypes in the North Indian population. *Hum. Immunol.* **63:** 24–29.

43. Mehra N.K., R. Jaini, R. Rajalingam, A. Balamurugan, *et al.* 2001. Molecular diversity of HLA-A*02 in Asian Indians: predominance of A*0211. *Tissue Antigen* **57**: 502–507.

44. Cai, J., P.I. Terasaki, N. Anderson, *et al.* 2009. Intact HLA not beta2m-free heavy chain-specific HLA class I antibodies are predictive of graft failure. *Transplantation* **88**: 226–230.

45. Zoet Y. M., S. H. Brand-Schaaf, D. L. Roelen, *et al.* 2011. Challenging the golden standard in defining donor-specific antibodies: does the solid phase assay meet the expectations? *Tissue Antigen* **77**: 225–228.

46. Roelen, D.L., I.I. Doxiadis & F.H. Claas. 2012. Detection and clinical relevance of donor specific HLA antibodies: a matter of debate. *Transpl. Int.* **25**: 604–610.

47. Amico, P., G. Honger, M. Mayr, *et al.* 2009. Clinical relevance of pretransplant donor-specific HLA antibodies detected by single-antigen flow-beads. *Transplantation* **87**: 1681–1688.

48. Otten, H.G., M.C. Verhaar, H.P.E. Borst, *et al.* 2012. Pretransplant donor-specific HLA class-I and -II antibodies are associated with an increased risk for kidney graft failure. *Am. J. Transplant.* **12**: 1618–1623.

49. Jolly, E.C., T. Key, H. Rasheed, *et al.* 2012. Preformed donor HLA-DP-specific antibodies mediate acute and chronic antibody-mediated rejection following renal transplantation. *Am. J. Transplant.* **12**: 2845–2848.

50. Panigrahi, A., N. Gupta, J.A. Siddiqui, *et al.* 2007. Posttransplant development of MICA and anti-HLA antibodies is associated with acute rejection episodes and renal allograft loss. *Hum. Immunol.* **68**: 362–367.

51. Susal, C., B. Dohler & G. Opelz. 2009. Presensitized kidney graft recipients with HLA class I and II antibodies are at increased risk for graft failure: a collaborative transplant study report. *Hum. Immunol.* **70**: 569–573.

52. Taylor, C.J., V. Kosmoliaptsis, D.M. Summers & J.A. Bradley. 2009. Back to the future: application of contemporary technology to long-standing questions about the clinical relevance of human leukocyte antigen-specific alloantibodies in renal transplantation. *Hum. Immunol.* **70**: 563–568.

53. Samaniego, M., J. Mezrich, J. Torrealba, *et al.* 2006. C4d positive acute antibody-mediated rejection due to anti HLA-DP antibody: a tale of one patient and a review of the University of Wisconsin experience. *Clin. Transpl.* 503–507.

54. Goral, S., E.L. Prak, Kearns, *et al.* 2008. Preformed donor directed anti-HLA DP antibodies may be an impediment to successful kidney transplantation. *Nephrol. Dial. Transplant.* **23**: 390–392.

55. Thaunat, O., W. Hanf, V. Dubois, *et al.* 2009. Chronic humoral rejection mediated by anti HLA-DP alloantibodies-insights into the role of epitope sharing in donor specific and non donor specific alloantibodies generation. *Transpl. Immunol.* **20**: 209–211.

56. Singh, P., B.W. Colombe, G.C. Francos, *et al.* 2010. Acute humoral rejection in a zero mismatch deceased donor renal transplant due to an antibody to an HLA-DP. *Transplantation* **90**: 220–221.

57. Gilbert, M., S. Paul, G. Perrat, *et al.* 2011. Impact of pretransplant human leukocyte antigen-C and -DP antibodies on kidney graft outcome. *Transplant. Pro.* **43**: 3412–3414.

58. Willicombe, M., C. Roufosse, P. Brookes, *et al.* 2011. Antibody-mediated rejection after alemtuzumab induction: incidence, risk factors and predictors of poor outcome. *Transplantation* **92**: 176–182.

59. Lee, P.C., M. Ozawa, C.J. Hung, *et al.* 2009. Eighteen-year follow-up of a retrospective study of HLA antibody on kidney graft survival. *Transplant. Proc.* **41**: 121–123.

60. Willicombe, M., P. Brookes, R. Sergeant, *et al.* 2012. De novo DQ donor-specific antibodies are associated with a significant risk of antibody-mediated rejection and transplant glomerulopathy. *Transplantation* **94**: 172–177.

61. Gibbs, V.C., D.M. Wood & M.R. Garovoy. 1985. The response of cultured human kidney capillary endothelium to immunologic stimuli. *Hum. Immunol.* **14**: 259–269.

62. Piazza, A., E. Poggi, L. Borrelli, *et al.* 2001. Impact of donor-specific antibodies on chronic rejection occurrence and graft loss in renal transplantation: posttransplant analysis using flow cytometric techniques. *Transplantation* **71**: 1106–1112.

63. Crespo, M., M. Pascual, N. Tolkoff-Rubin, *et al.* 2001. Acute humoral rejection in renal allograft recipients: I. Incidence, serology and clinical characteristics. *Transplantation* **71**: 652–658.

64. Zhang, Q., L.W. Liang, D.W. Gjertson, *et al.* 2005. Development of posttransplant antidonor HLA antibodies is associated with acute humoral rejection and early graft dysfunction. *Transplantation* **79**: 591–598.

65. Roelen, D.L., J. van Bree, M.D. Witvliet, *et al.* 1994. IgG antibodies against an HLA antigen are associated with activated cytotoxic T cells against this antigen, IgM are not. *Transplantation* **57**: 1388–1392.

66. Matinlauri, I.H., L.E. Kyllonen, B.H. Eklund, *et al.* 2004. Weak humoral posttransplant alloresponse after well-HLA-matched cadaveric kidney transplantation. *Transplantation* **78**: 198–204.

67. Yabu, J., J. Higgins, G. Chen, *et al.* 2011. C1q-fixing human leukocyte antigen antibodies are specific for predicting transplant glomerulopathy and late graft failure after kidney transplantation. *Transplantation* **91**: 342–347.

68. Sutherland, S.M., G. Chen, F.A. Sequeira, *et al.* 2011. Complement-fixing donor specific antibodies identified by a novel C1q assay are associated with allograft loss. *Pediatr. Transplant.* **16**: 12–17.

69. Chen, G., F. Sequeira & D.B. Tyan. 2011. Novel C1q assay reveals a clinically relevant subset of human leukocyte antigen antibodies independent of immunoglobulin G strength on single antigen beads. *Hum. Immunol.* **72**: 849–858.

70. Jordan, S.C., H.K. Yap, R.S. Sakai, *et al.* 1988. Hyperacute allograft rejection mediated by anti-vascular endothelial cell antibodies with a negative monocyte crossmatch. *Transplantation* **46**: 585–587.

71. Kalil, J., L. Guilherme, J. Neumann, *et al.* 1989. Humoral rejection in two HLA-identical living related donor kidney transplants. *Transplant. Proc.* **21**: 711–713.

72. Harmer, A.W., D. Haskard, C.G. Koffman & K.I. Welsh. 1990. Novel antibodies associated with unexplained loss of renal allografts. *Transpl. Int.* **3**: 66–69.

73. Sumitran-Karuppan, S., G. Tyden, F. Reinholt, *et al.* 1997. Hyperacute rejections of two consecutive renal allografts and early loss of the third transplant caused by non-HLA

antibodies specific for endothelial cells. *Transpl. Immunol.* **5:** 321–327.

74. Sun, Q., Z. Liu, J. Chen, *et al.* 2008. Circulating anti-endothelial cell antibodies are associated with poor outcome in renal allograft recipients with acute rejection. *Clin. J. Am. Soc. Nephrol.* **3:** 1479–1486.

75. Ronda, C., S.C.P. Borba, S.C.P. Ferreira, *et al.* 2011. Non-human leukocyte antigen antibodies reactive with endothelial cells could be involved in early loss of renal allografts. *Transplant. Proc.* **43:** 1345–1348.

76. Dragun, D., D.N. Muller, J.H. Brasen, *et al.* 2005. Angiotensin II type 1-receptor activating antibodies in renal-allograft rejection. *N. Engl. J. Med.* **352:** 558–569.

77. Jurcevic, S., M.E. Ainsworth, A. Pomerance, *et al.* 2001. Antivimentin antibodies are an independent predictor of transplant-associated coronary artery disease after cardiac transplantation. *Transplantation* **71:** 886–892.

78. Sumitran-Holgersson, S., H.E. Wilczek, J. Holgersson & K. Soderstrom. 2002. Identification of the non classical HLA molecules, MICA, as targets for humoral immunity associated with irreversible rejection of kidney allografts. *Transplantation* **74:** 268–277.

79. Joosten, S.A., Y.W. Sijpkens, V.V. Ham, *et al.* 2005. Antibody response against the glomerular basement membrane protein a grin in patients with transplant glomerulopathy. *Am. J. Transplant.* **5:** 383–393.

80. Jackson, A.M., D.P. Lucas, J.K. Melancon & N.M. Desai. 2011. Clinical Relevance and Ig G subclass determination of non-HLA antibodies identified using endothelial cell precursors isolated from donor blood. *Transplantation* **92:** 54–60.

81. Zwirner, N.W., M.A. Fernandez-Vina & P. Stastny. 1998. MICA, a new polymorphic HLA related antigen, is expressed mainly by keratinocytes, endothelial cells, and monocytes. *Immunogenetic* **47:** 139–148.

82. Mizutani, K., P. Terasaki, A. Rosen, *et al.* 2005. Serial ten-year follow-up of HLA and MICA antibody production prior to kidney graft failure. *Am. J. Transplant.* **5:** 2265–2272.

83. Zou, Y., F.M. Heinemann, H. Grosse-Wilde, *et al.* 2006. Detection of anti-MICA antibodies in patients awaiting kidney transplantation, during the post-transplant course, and in eluates from rejected kidney allografts by Luminex flow cytometry. *Hum. Immunol.* **67:** 230–237.

84. Zou, Y., P. Stastny, C. Susal, *et al.* 2007. Antibodies against MICA antigens and kidney-transplant rejection. *N. Engl. J. Med.* **357:** 1293–1300.

85. Zwirner, N.W., C.Y. Marcos, F. Mirbaha, *et al.* 2000. Identification of MICA as a new polymorphic alloantigen recognized by antibodies in sera of organ transplant recipients. *Hum. Immunol.* **61:** 917–924.

86. Lemy, A., M. Andrien, K.M. Wissing, *et al.* 2010. Major histocompatibility complex class I chain-related antigen A antibodies: sensitizing events and impact on renal graft outcomes. *Transplantation* **90:** 168–174.

87. Kato, M., T. Kinukawa, R. Hattori, *et al.* 2006. Does MICA influence acute rejection in kidney transplantation? *Clin. Transpl.* **20:** 389–393.

88. Narayan, S., E.W. Tsai, Q. Zhang, *et al.* 2011. Acute rejection associated with donor-specific anti-MICA antibody in a highly sensitized pediatric renal transplant recipient. *Pediatr. Transplant.* **15:** E1–E7.

89. Becker, Y.T., B.N. Becker, J.D. Pirsch & H.W. Sollinger. 2004. Rituximab as treatment for refractory kidney transplant rejection. *Am. J. Transplant.* **4:** 996–1001.

90. Faguer, S., N. Kamar, C. Guilbeaud-Frugier, *et al.* 2007. Rituximab therapy for acute humoral rejection after kidney transplantation. *Transplantation* **83:** 1277–1280.

91. Trivedi, H.L., P.I. Terasaki, A. Feroz, *et al.* 2009. Abrogation of anti- HLA antibodies via proteasome inhibition. *Transplantation* **87:** 1555–1561.

92. Walsh, R.C., J.J. Everly, P. Brailey, *et al.* 2010. Proteasome inhibitor based primary therapy for antibody-mediated renal allograft rejection. *Transplantation* **89:** 277–284.

93. Duquesnoy, R.J. 2011. Antibody reactive epitope determination with HLAMatchmaker and its clinical applications. *Tissue Antigens* **77:** 525–534.

ANNALS OF THE NEW YORK ACADEMY OF SCIENCES

Issue: *Translational Immunology in Asia-Oceania*

Th2-type innate immune responses mediated by natural helper cells

Shigeo Koyasu[1,2] and Kazuyo Moro[1,2,3]

[1]Department of Microbiology and Immunology, Keio University School of Medicine, Tokyo, Japan. [2]Laboratory for Immune Cell System, RIKEN Research Center for Allergy and Immunology, Yokohama, Japan. [3]PRESTO, JST, Tokyo, Japan

Address for correspondence: Shigeo Koyasu, Department of Microbiology and Immunology, Keio University School of Medicine, 35 Shinanomachi, Shinjuku-ku, Tokyo 160-8582, Japan. koyasu@z3.keio.jp

Natural helper (NH) cells are a newly identified innate lymphocyte population that responds to a combination of interleukin (IL)-2 and either IL-25 or IL-33 to produce large amounts of T helper cell type 2 (Th2) cytokines. NH cells have been identified in fat-associated lymphoid clusters (FALCs), produce Th2 cytokines constitutively without any stimulation, and support the self-renewal of B1 cells and IgA production by B cells. Large amounts of IL-5 and IL-13 produced upon helminth infection or in response to IL-33 can induce eosinophilia and goblet cell hyperplasia in the lung and intestine; these cytokines, which activate NH cells, play important roles in antihelminth immunity and allergic diseases such as asthma.

Keywords: natural helper cells; innate immunity; cytokine; IL-5; helminth

Introduction

The cooperation of innate and adaptive immune responses is critical for protective immunity against infection.[1] Distinct types of helper T (Th) cells play different roles in adaptive immune responses. Th1 cells play an important role in the control of intracellular microbes by producing interferon-γ (IFN-γ) to activate macrophages and cytotoxic T lymphocytes.[2] Th2 cell–derived cytokines are important for the activation of mast cells, eosinophils, and goblet cells during anti-helminth immunity.[2] Th17 cells activate epithelial cells to produce antimicrobial peptides and recruit neutrophils to combat extracellular bacterial infection.[3] Since it takes several days to establish antigen-specific Th cell responses, innate immune responses are critical for limiting the early growth and expansion of invading microbes.

In addition to two prototypic innate lymphocyte populations, namely classical natural killer (NK) and lymphoid tissue inducer (LTi) cells, recent studies have identified various types of innate lymphocytes. These include NK receptor–positive LTi cells,[4] LTi cells that produce interleukin (IL)-17 and IL-22,[5] and Th2-type innate lymphocytes, such as natural helper (NH) cells.[6] The transcription factor Id2 is essential for the differentiation of all innate lymphocytes, suggesting the presence of a common progenitor population. Like Th cell subsets in adaptive immune responses, NK, LTi, and NH cells play distinct roles in innate immune responses by producing Th1, Th17, and Th2 cytokines, respectively[7,8] (Table 1). Cooperation between innate lymphocytes and antigen-specific T and B cells is likely important for efficient protective immunity against various microbial infections, although excessive responses can result in inflammatory responses that are harmful to the host (Fig. 1).

First reported in 2010, a Lin⁻Thy-1⁺IL-7R⁺GATA3⁺ lymphocyte subset that was retinoic acid receptor–related orphan receptor γ (RORγ) independent but dependent on both Id2 and IL-7 and produced Th2 cytokines (most notably IL-5 and IL-13) was variously named *NH cells*,[9] *nuocytes*,[10] or *innate helper type 2* (Ih2) cells[11] by different research groups. NH cells were identified in naive animals, while nuocytes and Ih2 cells were observed in mice either after cytokine administration or during helminth infection. Although the

doi: 10.1111/nyas.12106

Table 1. Comparison between NK, LTi-related, and NH cells

| Characteristics | Cells | | | | | |
| | NK | NKR$^+$ LTi | | NKR$^-$ LTi | | NH |
		RORγ^+	RORγ^-	Adult	Fetal	
Cytokines produced	IFN-γ	IFN-γ, IL-17	IL-17, IL-22	IL-17, IL-22	TNF-α, LTα, LTβ	IL-5, IL-6, IL-13
Localization	All lymphoid tissue	Intestine	Intestine	All lymphoid tissue	Lymph node anlagen	Adipose tissue, lung
Group[a]	1	1	3	3		2

[a]The innate lymphoid cells are categorized into three groups.[66]

relationship between the cells is currently unclear, NH cells, nuocytes, and Ih2 cells share similar characteristics.

Cytokines that induce Th2-type innate immune responses

Recent studies have shed light on the role of epithelial cells in the regulation of immune responses. Epithelial cell–derived IL-25 and IL-33 have been implicated in regulating Th2-type innate immune responses. IL-17E, also known as IL-25, is a member of the IL-17 family,[12] but unlike other IL-17 family members, IL-17E induces Th2 immune responses.[13] Compared with wild-type mice, transgenic mice expressing either mouse or human IL-25 produce increased levels of serum IL-5 and IL-13 and have eosinophilia.[14, 15] IL-25 was originally considered to be a Th2 cytokine produced by Th2 cells,[12] but further studies have shown that this cytokine is also produced by epithelial cells, such as gut epithelial cells in mice infected with *Nippostrongylus brasiliensis*[16] and lung epithelial cells in mice infected with *Aspergillus fumigatus*.[13] Mast cells activated through FcεRI also produce IL-25.[17]

The importance of IL-25 to Th2 immune responses was demonstrated using IL-25–deficient mice, which are unable to elicit a Th2 response upon *Trichuris muris* infection and thus cannot control infection.[18] Similarly, the expulsion of *N. brasiliensis* is significantly delayed in IL-25–deficient mice.[19] Administration of recombinant IL-25 leads to the expulsion of *N. brasiliensis* even in Rag1–deficient mice that lack both T and B cells, suggesting a pivotal role for the innate immune response in this process. IL-25 has been shown to activate NKT cells[20] and c-Kit$^+$ non-T non-B cells.[19, 21]

IL-33, a member of the IL-1 family, binds to a heterodimeric receptor formed by T1/ST2 and IL-RAP.[22] IL-33 is expressed by a variety of cells, including fibroblasts, epithelial cells, and endothelial cells,[22–24] and is localized in the nucleus.[25] Although IL-33 can be cleaved by caspase 1 *in vitro*,[26] it is thought that caspases 3 and 7 inactivate IL-33 by cleaving it at the IL-1–like domain during apoptosis.[27, 28] In contrast, full-length IL-33, as released from cells upon necrotic death, functions as an alarmin to stimulate a variety of cells.[27] Similar alarmins include HMGB-1[29] and IL-1α,[30] which are also present in the nucleus and are released upon cellular damage. IL-33R is expressed by various types of cells, including Th2 cells,[31] mast cells,[32] basophils,[33, 34] NK cells, and NKT cells.[33, 35] IL-33 induces the production of IL-5 and IL-13 from Th2 cells,[31] basophils,[36] and mast cells;[37] and administration of IL-25 or IL-33 to mice induces the rapid production of Th2 cytokines, including as IL-5 and IL-13, independently of T or B cells.[12, 13, 38] These data suggest that Th2 cytokine–producing innate lymphocytes are regulated by epithelial cell–derived cytokines.

The remainder of this article documents the discovery and characterization of these Th2 cytokine-producing innate lymphocytes, NH cells.

NH cells and Th2-type immune responses

NH cells were identified in lymphoid clusters in adipose tissues.[9] Specifically, a previously unrecognized γ_c-dependent lymphoid structure was noted along the blood vessels in mouse and human mesenteries within adipose tissue in the peritoneal cavity.[9] These lymphoid clusters were named *fat-associated lymphoid clusters* (FALCs); cells in FALCs are in direct contact with ambient adipocytes, and no

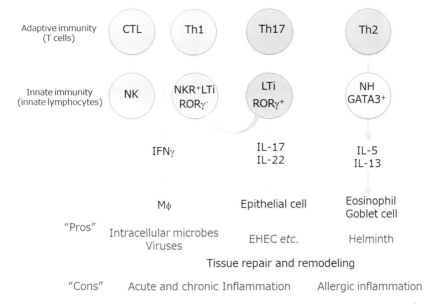

Figure 1. Role of adaptive and innate lymphocytes in infectious immunity and inflammation. NK cells, RORγ⁺ LTi–related cells, and Th2-type innate lymphocytes, such as NH cells, play distinct roles in innate immune responses by producing Th1, Th17, and Th2 cytokines, respectively (shown by straight arrows), before antigen-specific helper T (Th) cells are established. NK-receptor (NKR) expressing LTi-related cells that lost the expression of RORγ produce IFNγ (shown by an arch-type arrow), but have little cytotoxic activity, implying that NK cells and RORγ⁻ LTi–related cells in innate immunity correspond to cytotoxic T cells (CTL) and Th1 cells, respectively. These cells play important, beneficial roles in infectious immunity (pros), while they are also involved in various inflammatory responses, which are sometimes harmful to the hosts (cons).

fibrous capsule is present around FALCs. FALCs are also present in visceral adipose tissues around the kidney and genitalia, and are structurally similar to the milky spot in the omentum, which is considered a gateway of cells between the circulation and the peritoneal cavity.[39] However, unlike the milky spot,[40] no obvious T and B cell zones or germinal center structures are observed in FALCs.[9] FALCs are present in RORγ-deficient and *aly/aly* mice, suggesting that the differentiation pathway of FALCs is distinct from those of lymph nodes or Peyer's patches involving LTi cells.[41]

As in lymph nodes, T and B cells, macrophages, and dendritic cells (DCs) are present in FALCs. In addition, a cell population expressing c-Kit, Sca-1, IL-2R, IL-7R, and IL-33R, but no lineage (Lin) markers, was found to make up 20–40% of total cells (as measured by flow cytometry) in the lymphocytes.[9] Such cells were found to be abundant in visceral adipose tissues but not in subcutaneous fat tissue. In addition, these cells were present in $Rag2^{-/-}$ and *nu/nu* mice but absent from $Id2^{-/-}$, $\gamma_c^{-/-}$, and $Il7^{-/-}$ mice, indicating that they were likely of lymphoid lineage, with their differ-

entiation dependent on IL-7. *In vitro* experiments showed that IL-7 supported the survival of the cells and IL-2 induced their proliferation without changing their surface phenotype. A cell population expressing c-Kit and IL-7Rα is also present in human FALCs; Giemsa staining viewed by electron microscopy showed that these cells have characteristics of lymphoid cells. Since the mouse-derived innate lymphocytes proliferated in response to IL-2 and exhibited innate-type helper functions by producing Th2 cytokines, they were named NH cells.[9]

NH cells were not found in peripheral lymph nodes (LNs), including mesenteric lymph nodes (mLNs), which is distinct from nuocytes and Ih2 cells that are induced in lymph nodes upon helminth infection, as well as administration of IL-25.[10,11] In addition to Thy-1 and IL-7R, NH cells isolated from FALCs were found to express c-Kit, Sca-1, CD25, CD44, CD69, α₄β₇, ICOS, IL-17RB (IL-25R), and T1/ST2 (IL-33R), but not MHC class II, Flt3, or conventional lineage markers. Additional experiments have shown that NH cells express Id2 and GATA3, but lack RORγ.

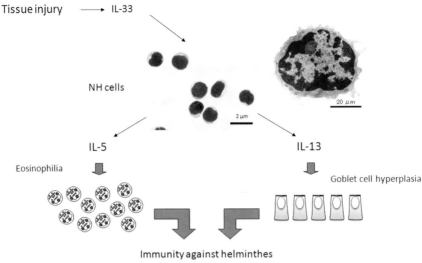

Immunity against helminthes
Pathophysiology of allergic diseases

Figure 2. A schematic model for the role of NH cells in the innate immune response against helminth infection as well as in the pathophysiology of allergic diseases. Helminth infection, as well as invasion of allergens, results in tissue damage, leading to the release of IL-33 from epithelial and endothelial cells. IL-33 acts on NH cells to produce large amounts of IL-5 and IL-13, which induce eosinophilia and goblet cell hyperplasia, respectively. These reactions are critical in host defense against helminth infection, and on the other hand, harmful for the host during allergic responses.

Differential expression of transcription factors discriminates NH cells from LTi or LTi-related innate lymphocytes. NH cells have been observed in the bone marrow (BM), where their expression of c-Kit is very low,[42] and in the lungs of naive mice.[43–47] A notable characteristic of NH cells is their ability to produce IL-5, IL-6, and IL-13 constitutively.[48,49] IL-5 is a critical growth factor for B1 cells, which are abundant in the peritoneal cavity and play an important role in innate-type immune responses by producing natural antibodies.[50,51] Indeed, NH cells have been shown to support the production of IgA from B cells and self-renewal of B1 cells, indicating that NH cells have helper functions under steady-state conditions.[9]

Upon activation with IL-33, NH cells have been shown to produce large amounts of IL-5 and IL-13. Five thousand NH cells can produce microgram amounts of IL-5 and IL-13 in response to IL-33 during a 5-day culture period,[9] much higher amounts than that produced by mast cells,[32] basophils,[33,34] or polarized Th2 cells.[31] IL-25 alone is unable to activate NH cells, but a combination of IL-2 and IL-25 can activate them to produce IL-5 and IL-13. It is notable that NH cells express mRNA for IL-4, although IL-4 protein is not induced by

IL-33 or by IL-2 and IL-25 stimulation. To date, only a combination of phorbol 12-myristate 13-acetate and ionomycin has been shown to stimulate NH cells to produce IL-4 at the protein level. It is possible that there is an epigenetic and/or posttranscriptional regulatory mechanisms for IL-4 expression in NH cells, and that NH cells may therefore produce IL-4 under certain circumstances.

NH cells have been shown to play an important role in innate immune responses against helminth infection.[52] Infection with *N. brasiliensis* is a model for the migratory pathway of human hookworm, which infects via a subcutaneous route, enters the vasculature, migrates to the lungs, molts, penetrates the alveoli, and ascends to the trachea where the worms are swallowed to complete maturation in the small intestine.[53,54] Th2 cytokines such as IL-13, which is essential for goblet cell hyperplasia and mucin production, are critical for the clearance of adult worms.[54–56]

Although $Il4^{-/-}$ mice exhibit an altered Th2 response, they can expel the *N. brasiliensis* worms and prevent infection,[57] unlike $Il13^{-/-}$ mice, which have impaired goblet cell hyperplasia.[55,58] Mice deficient in both γc and RAG2 ($\gamma_c^{-/-}$ $Rag2^{-/-}$ mice), and thus lacking NH cells, produce neither IL-5 nor

IL-13 and exhibit impaired eosinophilia in the lungs and impaired goblet cell hyperplasia in the intestine upon *N. brasiliensis* infection. Intranasal administration of IL-33 has been shown to induce NH cells in the lung and bronchoalveolar lavage (BAL) fluid associated with eosinophilia, whereas IL-25 is less potent than IL-33 (see Refs. 59 and 60; and unpublished observations, S. Koyasu and K. Moro); administration of IL-33 fails to induce IL-5 and IL-13 production in $\gamma_c^{-/-}$ *Rag2*$^{-/-}$ mice. However, adoptive transfer of NH cells isolated from FALCs can restore both eosinophilia and goblet cell hyperplasia and production of IL-5 and IL-13.

Together, these data indicate that NH cells likely contribute to the early production of IL-5 and IL-13 to induce eosinophilia and goblet cell hyperplasia, responses that play pivotal roles in antihelminth innate immunity.

Perspectives

Since IL-5 and IL-13 are critical factors in the induction of eosinophilia and goblet cell hyperplasia, respectively, and since these two processes are involved in both antihelminth immunity and the pathogenesis of allergic diseases, such as asthma and allergic diarrhea, Th2-type innate lymphocytes likely play important roles in these allergic diseases (Fig. 2).

NH cells do not respond to Toll-like receptor (TLR) ligands, such as lipopolysaccharide (LPS), or to lectins, such as concanavalin A (see Ref. 9, and unpublished observations, S. Koyasu and K. Moro). It is currently unknown whether Th2-type innate lymphocytes directly respond to allergens or microbial/parasitic antigens. It also remains to be shown whether the triggering of NH cells depends on cellular damage or on allergen stimulation of epithelia, or whether NH cells directly recognize foreign antigens.

In addition to their roles in allergic diseases and protection against helminth infection, NH cells may have additional roles, as FALC are present in adipose tissues. Accumulating evidence has demonstrated the importance of interactions between adipocytes and immune cells in the regulation of adipose tissue homeostasis. For example, impaired regulation during pathogenic conditions, such as obesity, may result in inflammatory responses in adipose tissues, leading to insulin resistance.[61] A subset of macrophages, the M1 macrophage, is involved in adipose tissue inflammation,[61,62] and although IL-33 can induce the M2 subset of macrophages, high levels of Th2 cytokines induce M1 macrophages.[63–65] In future studies, it will be important to elucidate the functions of NH cells in adipose tissue inflammation.

Acknowledgments

The author thanks his collaborators and the members of his laboratory. This work was supported by a Grant-in-Aid for Scientific Research (S) (No. 22229004) to S.K., a Grant-in-Aid for Young Scientist (A) (no. 22689013) to K.M. from the Japan Society for the Promotion of Science, a Grant-in-Aid for Scientific Research on Innovative Areas (No. 23118526) to K.M. from the Ministry of Education, Culture, Sports, Science and Technology, Japan, and PRESTO to K.M. from the Japan Science and Technology Agency.

Conflicts of interest

S.K. is a consultant for Medical and Biological Laboratories, Co. Ltd.

References

1. Zygmunt, B. & M. Veldhoen. 2011. T helper cell differentiation more than just cytokines. *Adv. Immunol.* **109:** 159–196.
2. Mossman, T.R. & R.L. Coffman. 1989. TH1 and TH2 cells: different patterns of lymphokine secretion lead to different functional properties. *Annu. Rev. Immunol.* **7:** 145–173.
3. Ouyang, W., J.K. Kolls & Y. Zheng. 2008. The biological functions of T helper 17 effector cytokines in inflammation. *Immunity* **28:** 454–467.
4. Mortha, A. & A. Diefenbach. 2011. Natural killer cell receptor-expressing innate lymphocytes: more than just NK cells. *Cell Mol. Life Sci.* **68:** 3541–3555.
5. Spits, H. & J.P. Di Santo. 2011. The expanding family of innate lymphoid cells: regulators and effectors of immunity and tissue remodeling. *Nat. Immunol.* **12:** 21–27.
6. Koyasu, S. & K. Moro. 2011. Innate Th2-type immune responses and the natural helper cell, a newly identified lymphocyte population. *Curr. Opin. Allergy Clin. Immunol.* **11:** 109–114.
7. Koyasu, S. & K. Moro. 2012. Natural "helper" cells in the lung: good or bad help? *Immunity* **36:** 317–319.
8. Koyasu, S. & K. Moro. 2012. Role of innate lymphocytes in infection and inflammation. *Front. Immunol.* **3:** 101.
9. Moro, K., T. Yamada, M. Tanabe, *et al.* 2010. Innate production of Th2 cytokines by adipose tissue-associated c-Kit$^+$Sca-1$^+$ lymphoid cells. *Nature* **463:** 540–544.
10. Neill, D.R., S.H. Wong, A. Bellosi, *et al.* 2010. Nuocytes represent a new innate effector leukocyte that mediates type-2 immunity. *Nature* **464:** 1367–1370.
11. Price, A.E., H.E. Liang, B.M. Sullivan, *et al.* 2010. Systemically dispersed innate IL-13-expressing cells in type 2 immunity. *Proc. Natl. Acad. Sci. USA* **107:** 11489–11494.

12. Fort, M.M., J. Cheung, D. Yen, *et al.* 2001. IL-25 induces IL-4, IL-5 & IL-13 and Th2-associated pathologies *in vivo*. *Immunity* **15**: 985–995.

13. Hurst, S.D., T. Muchamuel, D.M. Gorman, *et al.* 2002. New IL-17 family members promote Th1 or Th2 responses in the lung: *in vivo* function of the novel cytokine IL-25. *J. Immunol.* **169**: 443–453.

14. Kim, M.R., R. Manoukian, R. Yeh, *et al.* 2002. Transgenic overexpression of human IL-17E results in eosinophilia, B-lymphocyte hyperplasia & altered antibody production. *Blood* **100**: 2330–2340.

15. Pan, G., D. French, W. Mao, *et al.* 2001. Forced expression of murine IL-17E induces growth retardation, jaundice, a Th2-biased response & multiorgan inflammation in mice. *J. Immunol.* **167**: 6559–6567.

16. Angkasekwinai, P., H. Park, Y.H. Wang, *et al.* 2007. Interleukin 25 promotes the initiation of proallergic type 2 responses. *J. Exp. Med.* **204**: 1509–1517.

17. Ikeda, K., H. Nakajima, K. Suzuki, *et al.* 2003. Mast cells produce interleukin-25 upon FcεRI-mediated activation. *Blood* **101**: 3594–3596.

18. Owyang, A.M., C. Zaph, E.H. Wilson, *et al.* 2006. Interleukin 25 regulates type 2 cytokine-dependent immunity and limits chronic inflammation in the gastrointestinal tract. *J. Exp. Med.* **203**: 843–849.

19. Fallon, P.G., S.J. Ballantyne, N.E. Mangan, *et al.* 2006. Identification of an interleukin (IL)-25-dependent cell population that provides IL-4, IL-5 & IL-13 at the onset of helminth expulsion. *J. Exp. Med.* **203**: 1105–1116.

20. Terashima, A., H. Watarai, S. Inoue, *et al.* 2008. A novel subset of mouse NKT cells bearing the IL-17 receptor B responds to IL-25 and contributes to airway hyperreactivity. *J. Exp. Med.* **205**: 2727–2733.

21. Perrigoue, J.G., S.A. Saenz, M.C. Siracusa, *et al.* 2009. MHC class II-dependent basophil-CD4[+] T cell interactions promote T$_H$2 cytokine-dependent immunity. *Nat. Immunol.* **10**: 697–705.

22. Sanada, S., D. Hakuno, L.J. Higgins, *et al.* 2007. IL-33 and ST2 comprise a critical biomechanically induced and cardioprotective signaling system. *J. Clin. Invest.* **117**: 1538–1549.

23. Moussion, C., N. Ortega & J.P. Girard. 2008. The IL-1-like cytokine IL-33 is constitutively expressed in the nucleus of endothelial cells and epithelial cells *in vivo*: a novel 'alarmin'? *PLoS One* **3**: e3331.

24. Wood, I.S., B. Wang & P. Trayhurn. 2009. IL-33, a recently identified interleukin-1 gene family member, is expressed in human adipocytes. *Biochem. Biophys. Res. Commun.* **384**: 105–109.

25. Carrière, V., L. Roussel, N. Ortega, *et al.* 2007. IL-33, the IL-1-like cytokine ligand for ST2 receptor, is a chromatin-associated nuclear factor *in vivo*. *Proc. Natl. Acad. Sci. USA* **104**: 282–287.

26. Schmitz, J., A. Owyang, E. Oldham, *et al.* 2005. IL-33, an interleukin-1-like cytokine that signals via the IL-1 receptor-related protein ST2 and induces T helper type 2-associated cytokine. *Immunity* **23**: 479–490.

27. Cayrol, C. & J.P. Girard. 2009. The IL-1-like cytokine IL-33 is inactivated after maturation by caspase-1. *Proc. Natl. Acad. Sci. USA* **106**: 9021–9026.

28. Lüthi, A.U., S.P. Cullen, E.A. McNeela, *et al.* 2009. Suppression of interleukin-33 bioactivity through proteolysis by apoptotic caspases. *Immunity* **31**: 84–98.

29. Scaffidi, P., T. Misteli & M.E. Bianchi. 2002. Release of chromatin protein HMGB1 by necrotic cells triggers inflammation. *Nature* **418**: 191–195.

30. Cohen, I., P. Rider, Y. Carmi, *et al.* 2010. Differential release of chromatin-bound IL-1α discriminates between necrotic and apoptotic cell death by the ability to induce sterile inflammation. *Proc. Natl. Acad. Sci. USA* **107**: 2574–2579.

31. Xu, D., W.L. Chan, B.P. Leung, *et al.* 1998. Selective expression of a stable cell surface molecule on type 2 but not type 1 helper T cells. *J. Exp. Med.* **187**: 787–794.

32. Ali, S., M. Huber, C. Kollewe, *et al.* 2007. IL-1 receptor accessory protein is essential for IL-33-induced activation of T lymphocytes and mast cells. *Proc. Natl. Acad. Sci. USA* **104**: 18660–18665.

33. Smithgall, M.D., M.R. Comeau, B.R. Yoon, *et al.* 2008. IL-33 amplifies both Th1- and Th2-type responses through its activity on human basophils, allergen-reactive Th2 cells, iNKT and NK cells. *Int. Immunol.* **20**: 1019–1030.

34. Suzukawa, M., M. Iikura, R. Koketsu, *et al.* 2008. An IL-1 cytokine member, IL-33, induces human basophil activation via its ST2 receptor. *J. Immunol.* **181**: 5981–5989.

35. Bourgeois, E., L.P. Van, M. Samson, *et al.* 2009. The pro-Th2 cytokine IL-33 directly interacts with invariant NKT and NK cells to induce IFN-γ production. *Eur. J. Immunol.* **39**: 1046–1055.

36. Kondo, Y., T. Yoshimoto, K. Yasuda, *et al.* 2008. Administration of IL-33 induces airway hyperresponsiveness and goblet cell hyperplasia in the lungs in the absence of adaptive immune system. *Int. Immunol.* **20**: 791–800.

37. Ho, L.H., T. Ohno, K. Oboki, *et al.* 2007. IL-33 induces IL-13 production by mouse mast cells independently of IgE-FcεRI signals. *J. Leukoc. Biol.* **82**: 1481–1490.

38. Humphreys, N.E., D. Xu, M.R. Hepworth, *et al.* 2008. IL-33, a potent inducer of adaptive immunity to intestinal nematodes. *J. Immunol.* **180**: 2443–2449.

39. Cranshaw, M.L. & L.V. Leak. 1990. Milky spots of the omentum: a source of peritoneal cells in the normal and stimulated animal. *Arch. Histol. Cytol.* **53** (Suppl): 165–177.

40. Rangel-Moreno, J., J.E. Moyron-Quiroz, D.M. Carragher, *et al.* 2009. Omental milky spots develop in the absence of lymphoid tissue-inducer cells and support B and T cell responses to peritoneal antigens. *Immunity* **30**: 731–743.

41. Nishikawa, S., K. Honda, P. Vieira & H. Yoshida. 2003. Organogenesis of peripheral lymphoid organs. *Immunol. Rev.* **195**: 72–80.

42. Brickshawana, A., V.S. Shapiro, H. Kita & L.R. Pease. 2011. Lineage[−]Sca1[+]c-Kit[−]CD25[+] cells are IL-33-responsive type 2 innate cells in the mouse bone marrow. *J. Immunol.* **187**: 5795–5804.

43. Yang, Q., S.A. Saenz, D.A. Zlotoff, *et al.* 2011. Cutting edge: natural helper cells derive from lymphoid progenitors. *J. Immunol.* **187:** 5505–5509.

44. Monticelli, L.A., G.F. Sonnenberg, M.C. Abt, *et al.* 2011. Innate lymphoid cells promote lung-tissue homeostasis after infection with influenza virus. *Nat. Immunol.* **12:** 1045–1054.

45. Chang, Y.J., H.Y. Kim, L.A. Albacker, *et al.* 2011. Innate lymphoid cells mediate influenza-induced airway hyperreactivity independently of adaptive immunity. *Nat. Immunol.* **12:** 631–638.

46. Halim, T.Y., R.H. Krauss, A.C. Sun & F. Takei. 2012. Lung natural helper cells are a critical source of Th2 cell-type cytokines in protease allergen-induced airway inflammation. *Immunity* **36:** 451–463.

47. Ikutani, M., T. Yanagibashi, M. Ogasawara, *et al.* 2012. Identification of innate IL-5-producing cells and their role in lung eosinophil regulation and antitumor immunity. *J. Immunol.* **188:** 703–713.

48. Beagley, K.W., J.H. Eldridge, F. Lee, *et al.* 1989. Interleukins and IgA synthesis. Human and murine interleukin 6 induce high rate IgA secretion in IgA-committed B cells. *J. Exp. Med.* **169:** 2133–2148.

49. Sonoda, E., R. Matsumoto, Y. Hitoshi, *et al.* 1989. Transforming growth factor β induces IgA production and acts additively with interleukin 5 for IgA production. *J. Exp. Med.* **170:** 1415–1420.

50. Erickson, L.D., T.M. Foy & T.J. Waldschmidt. 2001. Murine B1 B cells require IL-5 for optimal T cell-dependent activation. *J. Immunol.* **166:** 1531–1539.

51. Martin, F. & J.F. Kearney. 2000. B-cell subsets and the mature preimmune repertoire. Marginal zone and B1 B cells as part of a "natural immune memory." *Immunol. Rev.* **175:** 70–79.

52. Koyasu, S., K. Moro, M. Tanabe & T. Takeuchi. 2010. Natural helper cells: a new player in the innate immune response against helminth infection. *Adv. Immunol.* **108:** 21–44.

53. Hotez, P.J., S. Brooker, J.M. Bethony, *et al.* 2004. Hookworm infection. *N. Engl. J. Med.* **351:** 799–807.

54. Maizels, R.M., E.J. Pearce, D. Artis, *et al.* 2009. Regulation of pathogenesis and immunity in helminth infections. *J. Exp. Med.* **206:** 2059–2066.

55. Urban, J.F. Jr., N.R. Steenhard, G.I. Solano-Aguilar, *et al.* 2007. Infection with parasitic nematodes confounds vaccination efficacy. *Vet. Parasitol.* **148:** 14–20.

56. Mohrs, K., A.E. Wakil, N. Killeen, *et al.* 2005. A two-step process for cytokine production revealed by IL-4 dual-reporter mice. *Immunity* **2:** 419–429.

57. Kopf, M., G. Le Gros, M. Bachmann, *et al.* 1993. Disruption of the murine IL-4 gene blocks Th2 cytokine responses. *Nature* **362:** 245–248.

58. McKenzie, G.J., P.G. Fallon, C.L. Emson, *et al.* 1999. Simultaneous disruption of interleukin (IL)-4 and IL-13 defines individual roles in T helper cell type 2-mediated responses. *J. Exp. Med.* **189:** 1565–1572.

59. Kim, H.Y., Y.J. Chang, S. Subramanian, *et al.* 2012. Innate lymphoid cells responding to IL-33 mediate airway hyperreactivity independently of adaptive immunity. *J. Allergy Clin. Immunol.* **129:** 216–227.

60. Wilhelm, C., K. Hirota, B. Stieglitz, *et al.* 2011. An IL-9 fate reporter demonstrates the induction of an innate IL-9 response in lung inflammation. *Nat. Immunol.* **12:** 1071–1077.

61. Suganami, T. & Y. Ogawa. 2010. Adipose tissue macrophages: their role in adipose tissue remodeling. *J. Leukoc. Biol.* **88:** 33–39.

62. Mantovani, A., A. Sica & M. Locati. 2005. Macrophage polarization comes of age. *Immunity* **23:** 344–346.

63. Murata, Y., A. Yamashita, T. Saito, *et al.* 2002. The conversion of redox status of peritoneal macrophages during pathological progression of spontaneous inflammatory bowel disease in Janus family tyrosine kinase 3$^{-/-}$ and IL-2 receptor γ$^{-/-}$ mice. *Int. Immunol.* **14:** 627–636.

64. Stolarski, B., M. Kurowska-Stolarska, P. Kewin, *et al.* 2010. IL-33 exacerbates eosinophil-mediated airway inflammation. *J. Immunol.* **185:** 3472–3480.

65. Hazlett, L.D., S.A. McClellan, R.P. Barrett, *et al.* 2010. IL-33 shifts macrophage polarization, promoting resistance against *Pseudomonas aeruginosa* keratitis. *Invest. Ophthalmol. Vis. Sci.* **51:** 1524–1532.

66. Spits, H., D. Artis, M. Colonna, *et al.* 2013. Innate lymphoid cells—a proposal for uniform nomenclature. *Nat. Rev. Immunol.* **13:** 145–149.

Ann. N.Y. Acad. Sci. ISSN 0077-8923

ANNALS OF THE NEW YORK ACADEMY OF SCIENCES

Issue: *Translational Immunology in Asia-Oceania*

A unique vaccine for control of fertility and therapy of advanced-stage terminal cancers ectopically expressing human chorionic gonadotropin

G. P. Talwar

Talwar Research Foundation, Neb Valley, New Delhi, India

Address for correspondence: Prof. G.P. Talwar, Talwar Research Foundation, E-8, Neb Valley, Neb Sarai, New Delhi-110068, India. gptalwar@gmail.com

Human chorionic gonadotropin (hCG) appears soon after fertilization of the egg and plays a critical role in implantation of the embryo leading to the beginning of pregnancy. Vaccines developed against hCG prevent pregnancy without impairment of ovulation and disturbance of menstrual regularity. A new recombinant vaccine hCGβ-LTB has been developed that is highly immunogenic in various strains of mice and intended for the control of fertility in women. An additional use of this vaccine is likely to be treatment of advanced-stage cancers that ectopically express hCG.

Keywords: HSD-TT; efficacy; hCGβ-LTB

Introduction

Human chorionic gonadotropin (hCG) is a highly interesting target for immunocontraception. It is not expressed by any organ of healthy men or nonpregnant healthy women. Thus, circulating antibodies against hCG do not react with any tissue of the body; hCG appears soon after fertilization of the egg. In the process of assisted reproduction, embryos resulting from *in vitro* fertilized eggs secrete hCG in the culture fluid before their transfer to the uterus.[1] hCG also plays a critical role in implantation of the embryo; for example, embryos exposed to anti-hCG antibodies fail to implant.[2] Thus, immunization against hCG, generating antibodies competent to block the bioactivity of hCG, achieves contraception without any pathological effect or contraindication; the reproductive system of the female operates normally. Women continue to produce leuteinizing hormone-releasing hormone (LHRH), which normally triggers the sequential secretion of follicle-stimulating hormone (FSH) and leuteinizing hormone (LH), to generate the egg and production and secretion of the sex steroids: estrogens and progesterone. The interception by anti-

bodies against hCG takes place only as and when hCG appears, which occurs soon after fertilization. Antibodies block implantation and thereby the onset of pregnancy. Among the many methods available currently for family planning, no other method matches the advantages and safety of immunocontraception by an anti-hCG vaccine. The additional merits of this approach are periodic intake (i.e., not daily) and privacy of use.

Vaccine production

Human chorionic gonadotropin or its subunits are not immunogenic per se in women. Flooded by this hormone during pregnancy, women nevertheless remain immunologically tolerant to it. To overcome the immunological tolerance, the β subunit of hCG (which confers on hCG its molecular identity, the α subunit of the hormone being identical to α of LH, TSH, and FSH) is conjugated to the carrier protein tetanus toxoid (TT). The conjugate hCG β-TT induces an anti-hCG antibody response in women.[3] The antibodies bind selectively to the hormone, inactivating its bioactivity. There is no risk of permanent autoreactivity as the response is completely reversible. The lack of interference in menstrual

doi: 10.1111/j.1749-6632.2012.06776.x

Ann. N.Y. Acad. Sci. 1283 (2013) 50–56 © 2013 New York Academy of Sciences.

regularity and reproductive hormones by vaccination has been demonstrated by trials not only in India, but also in Finland, Sweden, Chile, and Brazil under the auspices of the International Committee on Contraception Research (ICCR) of the Population Council (New York, NY).[4]

While linkage of hCG β with the carrier TT succeeded in inducing an antibody response to hCG, the titers of antibodies were low in three out of four women immunized. The next task was to improve the immunogenicity of the vaccine. To do that, we prepared a dimer of hCG β with the α subunit of ovine leuteinizing hormone (OLH). The idea was that the protein of ovine origin would be foreign to humans and hence antigenic. The β and α subunits, even of heterospecies origin, retain the intrinsic property of associating with each other noncovalently. Thus, a heterospecies dimer (HSD) of β-hCG and α-OLH was easily obtained. This was then linked to the carrier TT or DT (diptheria toxoid). HSD-TT proved to be more immunogenic than β-hCG-TT.[5] Furthermore HSD-TT–induced antibodies had better bioefficacy than those induced by β-hCG-TT. These were totally devoid of cross-reaction with hFSH and hTSH. Partial cross-reactivity existed with hLH, as hCG and hLH share large homologies of primary structure. However, partial cross-reaction with hLH did not prevent normal ovulation, as there is a sufficient reserve of hLH in the preovulatory surge to enable ovulation. Progesterone produced during the luteal phase was no doubt somewhat less. This however, contributed to the fertility control properties of the antigonadotropin vaccine, as demonstrated by Thau.[6]

Lack of contraindication of partial cross-reaction with hLH

Long-term (5–7 years) chronic toxicology studies were carried out in 63 female Rhesus monkeys to assess the safety of a vaccine that is partially cross-reactive with species LH.[7] The monkeys were hyperimmunized with ovine LH employing Freund's Complete Adjuvant and given boosters from time to time. The antibodies generated had cross-reaction with monkey LH. Monkeys became infertile, but they continued to ovulate. No abnormality was observed in pituitary function in spite of high-titer anti-LH antibodies in circulation over a long period.[7] Autopsies of several monkeys were performed to determine the possible damage that immune complexes may produce in kidneys and other organs. However, no such abnormalities were seen.[8]

Safety and efficacy of the HSD-TT/DT vaccine

After phase I safety trials of the HSD-TT/DT vaccine in many centers, indicating that the vaccine was devoid of any side effects,[9,10] the crucial phase II efficacy trials were undertaken in three major centers of India: the All India Institute of Medical Sciences, Postgraduate Institute of Medical Education and Research, Chandigarh, and Safdarjung Hospital, New Delhi. One hundred forty-eight sexually active married women of proven fertility with at least two children were enrolled for the trial. Many of these women were coming to these clinics for medical termination of pregnancy (MTP). The numerous family planning methods available free of charge were not suitable for them for one reason or the other. Women received three injections of 300 μg of the vaccine each at 6-week intervals as part of primary immunization. Thereafter, boosters were given when antibody titers declined. These were the first efficacy trials on any birth control vaccine in the world. Until then there was no formal proof that a vaccine that induced antibodies against hCG would indeed prevent women from becoming pregnant. Furthermore, the antibody titers required to confer pregnancy prevention were not known and had to be established. A putative threshold of 50 ng/mL bioneutralization capacity of hCG was initially fixed for testing. Intrauterine devices (IUDs) were used to prevent pregnancy in women during the period of primary immunization and then removed soon after the titers rose beyond 50 ng/mL. Ovulation was confirmed by measurement of luteal phase progesterone levels. Women enrolled in the trial engaged in sexual intercourse at least twice each week as per their statement. No pregnancies were recorded in women at antibody titers of 50 ng/mL bioneutralization capacity and above. The protection accorded by the vaccine was fairly high; only one pregnancy occurred in 1,224 cycles at and above 50 ng/mL. Figure 1 gives the profile of antibody titers in four women. They remained in trial for more than 2 years, receiving boosters as and when necessary. As is evident from Figure 1, all of the women continued to have regular periods. Eight women completed >30 cycles without becoming pregnant, 9 completed 24–29 cycles, 12 completed 18–23 cycles,

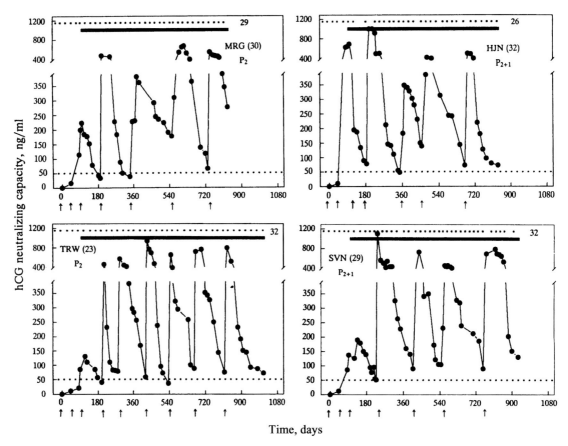

Figure 1. Antibody titers and menstrual record of four women immunized with 300 μg of HSD-TT/DT vaccine on days indicated by arrow. The solid line on the top represents the time period over which they were unprotected from becoming pregnant by IUCDs. Solid dots on the top indicate the days of menstrual periods. (Reproduced from Ref. 11.)

15 completed 12–17 cycles, and 21 subjects completed 6–11 cycles of continuous exposure to the possibility of pregnancy.[11] These results point to a fairly high efficacy of the anti-hCG vaccine to prevent pregnancy, without impairment of ovulation and derangement of menstrual regularity. Additionally, participants were enthusiastic to continue the vaccine. At the time the trial had to be concluded, some of the participants offered to pay for the vaccine to continue this mode of contraception.

The fact that in the absence of antibodies participants would have become pregnant is indicated by the 22 pregnancies that occurred in women at titers below 35 ng/mL.[11] Also, shown in Figure 2, is the case of a woman who was protected for 12 cycles and then decided to have a child, and thus did not receive a booster. She conceived readily in the cycle immediately following the antibody titers dropping below 35 ng/mL.

These trials are the first of their kind to provide evidence for the ability of anti-hCG antibodies to provide contraception without disturbance of the normal reproductive functions in women. Further, no permanent barrier is imposed, and women regain fertility on decline of antibody titers. The progeny born to women previously immunized with the anti-hCG vaccine were normal in their developmental landmarks and cognitive abilities.[12]

Revival of the vaccine

After a dormant period of 12 years, work on the anti-hCG vaccine was revived at the insistence of the Indo-U.S. Committee on Contraception and Child Health. We produced a recombinant vaccine with the consideration that it will be amenable to large-scale production by industry.

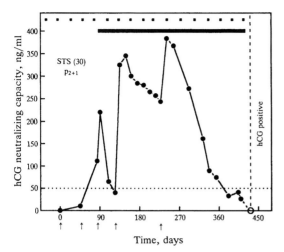

Figure 2. Regain of fertility on decline of antibodies. A 30-year-old subject (STS), with two gravidae and one elective abortion (P_{2+1}), on immunization with the vaccine remained protected from pregnancy for 12 cycles. In the absence of a booster injection, antibody titers declined and she became pregnant in the cycle starting on day 417. The extrapolated antibody titers at mid-cycle in the fertile month, shown by the dotted line, were <5 ng/mL. Reproduced from Ref. 11.

hCG-β was fused at the C-terminal end with the β subunit of heat labile enterotoxin of *E. coli* (LTB). hCG-β-LTB (Fig. 3) was expressed in *Pichia pastoris* to obtain the protein, which was adsorbed on alum, a permissible mode for human immunization.

Instead of oily adjuvants, we employed an autoclaved microorganism, *Mycobacterium indicus pranii* (MiP, previously coded as Mw), usable in saline suspension. Mw, now MiP,[13,14] was developed as an immunotherapeutic vaccine for multibacillary leprosy (for review, see Ref. 15). It is a nonpathogenic, fast-growing mycobacterium that acts as a potent adjuvant to boost antibody titers.[16] Although live MiP is a stronger inducer of immune responses, adjuvanticity is retained in the killed, autoclaved state.[17] *M. indicus pranii*, cross-reactive with both *M. leprae* and *M. tuberculosis*, is approved by the Drugs Controller General of India and also by the U.S. Food and Drug Administration in their orphan vaccine category. Clinicians have used MiP as an adjunct to multidrug regimen for treatment of category II, difficult-to-treat tuberculosis, with good results: faster AFB negativity and better cure results with much lower relapse rates.[18] Dipankar Nandi at the Indian Institute of Science Banglore has reported both prevention and regression of SP_2O

myleomas in mice by MiP.[19] Thus, MiP as adjuvant in the revived recombinant anti-hCG vaccine not only boosts anti-hCG antibody titers, in principle it may also help in the treatment of advanced-stage cancers ectopically expressing hCG.

High immunogenicity of the revived recombinant vaccine hCG-β-LTB

BalbC mice immunized with 2 µg of hCG-β-LTB-adsorbed alum plus MiP in saline induced antibodies in every mouse (100%, positivity of response), and the titers were well above the 50 ng/mL bioneutralization capacity; Figure 4 gives the geometric mean of titers at various time points after three primary immunizations and a booster on the 127th day, as well as the individual titers in each mouse.[20] In some mice, the titers went as high as 6,600 ng/mL. The antibody response was of long duration and well above the protective threshold of 50 ng/mL, as defined by previous phase II trials. It is, however, the anticipated clinical trials in women that will provide evidence on the higher immunogenicity of this vaccine compared to the vaccine used earlier.

As the immune response varies with the genetic makeup of the individual, it was appropriate to ask whether mice of other genetic strains also respond to the vaccine with titers above 50 ng/mL. Inbred mice of four other genetic strains, namely FVB, SJL, C3H, and C57Bl/6 were immunized with hCG-β-LTB. In each strain, three primary injections followed by a booster resulted in titers well above 50 ng/mL.[16] There was, however, variation in the magnitude of antibody response from strain to strain, as expected.

In summary, hCG-β-LTB recombinant vaccine has the potential for serving as a vaccine for control of fertility. It is currently in toxicology studies using a protocol developed by an expert committee of the Indian Council of Medical Research. If found safe, which is expected on grounds of the basic considerations that went into the choice of hCG as a target (it is not made by any tissue of nonpregnant females, hence antibodies would be free of cross-reactivity with all organs of the body), this vaccine would then go back to clinical trials for control of fertility.

Additional benefits of the hCG vaccine

A number of papers have appeared reporting the unexpected expression of human chorionic gonadotropin by a variety of cancers: expression

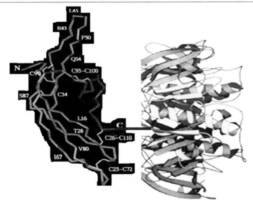

Figure 3. Conceptualized structure of LTB fused at the C-terminal end of hCG; the nnucleotide sequence of hCG-β is linked to the nucleotide sequence of LTB through linker GTCTAGA.

of alpha and beta genes of hCG in lung cancer,[21] urinary concentration of hCG as a prognostic marker in bladder cancer,[22] β-hCG as a prognostic marker in colorectal cancer,[23] elevation of free beta subunit of hCG and core beta fragment in the serum and urine of patients with malignant pancreatic and billiary diseases,[24] ectopic production of β-hCG by a maxillary squamous cell carcinoma,[25] and the prognostic significance of β-hCG in cervical carcinoma.[26] Invariably at the stage that ectopic expression of hCG/subunits takes place, the cancer is advanced and refractory to the currently available drugs. The prognosis of these patients of hCG-expressing tumors is poor with low survival rates. Tumors producing hCG are highly metastasizing and aggressive;[27] poor prognosis is reported in hCG-expressing bladder cancers, pancreatic exocrine tumors, and colorectal cancers.

Could the vaccine against hCG and or antibodies directed at hCG be of help in therapy of such patients? A number of cell lines have been developed from patients dying of such cancers. Anti-hCG antibodies have been shown to kill such cancer cells in culture.[28] The action occurs not only *in vitro* but also *in vivo*. Chago lung cancers in nude mice are inhibited in a dose-dependent manner by administration of antibodies against

hCG or its subunits.[29] Iles' group in the United Kingdom has started clinical trials in colorectal cancer patients. Early reports appearing in newspapers (http://www.dailymail.co.uk/health/article-1293927/Jab-hail-deadly-forms-cancer.html) report on "the shrinkage in size of the tumors and their invasiveness."

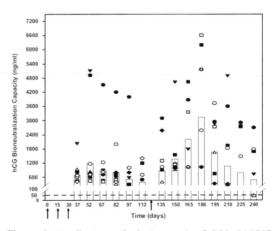

Figure 4. Bioeffective antibody titers against hCG in BALB/C mice immunized with hCG-β-LTB on alum + MiP. The symbols indicate the titers in each mouse at various time points; bars indicate the geometric means. 50 ng/mL is the titer required to prevent pregnancy in women as per previous phase II efficacy trails. Reproduced from Ref. 20.

Because the hCG/subunits expressed by such cancers are present on membranes of cells, anti-hCG antibodies labeled with radioisotopes can be employed for imaging of the metastasis and for targeted delivery of radiation.

It is not inconceivable that antibodies against hCG would not kill a given type of cancer cell, by themselves or in the presence of complement. We observed this in MOLT-4 T lymphoblastic leukemia cells. In such cases, antibodies against hCG that are linked to drugs could be employed to deliver drugs selectively to cancer cells. Our lab linked curcumin to a monoclonal anti-hCG antibody, demonstrating that the conjugate was effective in killing the MOLT-4 cells.[30]

Summary

Being an early product of the fertilized egg and playing a critical role in implantation and, thereby, in the start of pregnancy, hCG is potentially an excellent target for preventing pregnancy without any discernible side effects. In contrast to steroidal contraceptives that block ovulation, the hCG vaccine approach does not interrupt ovulation or normal production of sex hormones. Control of fertility is achieved without alteration of menstrual regularity.

The fact that a number of cancers of different origins ectopically produce hCG at an advanced stage opens up the additional potential of a highly immunogenic recombinant hCG vaccine for treatment of such terminal cancers.

Acknowledgments

I thank Renu Yadav for ably typing this manuscript and assistance in completing references. Also acknowledged are the precious contributions made by my PhD students, in particular, Shilpi Purswani and Hemant Vyas. I acknowledge with thanks the vital research Grants from the Department of Biotechnology, Government of India, and the Indian Council of Medical Research.

Conflicts of interest

The author declares no conflicts of interest.

References

1. Fishel, S.B., R.G. Edwards & C.J. Evans. 1984. Human chorionic gonadotropin secreted by pre-implantation embryos cultured in vitro. *Science* **223**: 816–818.

2. Hearn, J.P., A.A Gidley-Baird, J.K. Hodges & P.H. Summers. 1988. Embryonic signals during the pre-implantation period in primates. *J. Reprod. Fertil* 36(Suppl): 49–58.

3. Talwar, G.P., N.C. Sharma, S.K. Dubey, *et al.* 1976. Isoimmunization against human chorionic gonadotropin with conjugates of processed β subunit of the hormone and tetanus toxoid. *Proc. Natl. Acad. Sci USA* **73**: 218–222.

4. Nash, H., G.P. Talwar, S. Segal, *et al.* 1980. Observations on the antigenecity and clinical efficacy of a candidate antipregnancy vaccine: β subunit of hCG linked to tetanus toxoid. *Fertil. Steril.* **34**: 328–335.

5. Talwar, G.P., O. Singh & L.V. Rao. 1988. An improved immunogen for anti-human chorionic gonadotropin vaccine eliciting antibodies reactive with a conformation native to the hormone without cross-reaction with human follicle stimulating hormone and human thyroid stimulating hormone. *J. Reprod. Immunol* **14**: 203–212.

6. Thau, R.B., S.S. Witkin, M.G. Bond, *et al.* 1983. Effects of long term immunization against the beta subunit of ovine luteinizing hormone on circulating immune complex formation and on arterial changes in rhesus monkeys. *Am. J. Reprod. Immunol.* **3**: 83–88.

7. Thau, R.B., C.B. Wilson & K. Sundaram. 1987. Long-term immunization against β-Subunit of ovine luteinizing hormone (OLH- β) has no adverse effect on pituitary function in rhesus monkeys. *Am. J. Reprod. Immunol. Microbiol* **15**: 92–98.

8. Thau, R.B., M.G. Bond, S.S. Witkin, *et al.* 1986. Lack of toxicological effects following seven years of active immunization of rhesus monkeys with the β-subunit of OLH in *Immunological Approaches to Contraception & Promotion of Fertility*. G.P. Talwar, Ed. Plenum Press. New York, pp. 25–33.

9. Kharat, I., N.S. Nair, K. Dhall, *et al.* 1990. Analysis of menstrual records of women immunized with anti-hCG vaccines inducing antibodies partially cross-reactive with hLH. *Contraception* **41**: 293–299.

10. Talwar, G.P., V. Hingorani, S. Kumar, *et al.* 1990. Phase I clinical trials with three formulations of anti-human gonadotropin vaccine. *Contraception* **41**: 301–316.

11. Talwar, G.P., O. Singh, R. Pal, *et al.* 1994. A vaccine that prevents pregnancy in women. *Proc. Natl. Acad. Sci. USA* **91**: 8532–8536.

12. Singh, M., S.K. Das, S. Suri, *et al.* 1998. Regain of fertility and normality of progeny born at below protective threshold antibody titres in women immunised with the HSD-hCG vaccine. *Am. J. Reprod. Immunol* **39**: 395–398.

13. Talwar, G.P, N. Ahmad & V. Saini. 2008. The use of the name Mycobacterium W for the leprosy immunotherapeutic bacillus creates confusion with M.tuberculosis W (Beijing strain): a suggestion. *Infect. Genet. Evol.* **8**: 100–101.

14. Saini, V., S. Raghuvanshi, G.P. Talwar, *et al.* 2009. Polyphasic taxonomic analysis establishes Mycobacterium indicus pranii as a distinct species. *Plos One* **4**: e6263.

15. Talwar, G.P. 1999. An immunotherapeutic vaccine for multibacillary leprosy. *Int. Rev. Immunol.* **18**: 229–224.

16. Purswani, S., G.P. Talwar, R. Vohra, *et al.* 2011. Mycobacterium indicus pranii is a potent immunomodulator for a recombinant vaccine against human chorionic gonadotropin. *J. Reprod. Immuno* **91**: 24–30.

17. Gupta, A., G. Nishamol, J. Mani, *et al.* 2009. Immunogenecity and protective efficacy of Mycobacterium W against M. tuberculosis in mice immunised with live versus heat killed M.W. by the aerosol or parental route. *Infect. Immun.* **77:** 223–231.

18. Patel, N. & S.B. Tripathi. 2003. Improved cure rates in pulmonary tuberculosis category II (retreatment) with Mycobacterium w. *J. Indian. Med. Assoc.* **101:** 680–682.

19. Rakshit, S., M. Ponnusamy, S. Papanna, *et al.* 2012. Immunotherapeutic efficacy of *Mycobacterium indicus pranii* in eliciting anti-tumour T cell responses: critical roles of IFN-γ. *Int. J. Cancer* **130:** 865–875.

20. Puruswani, S. & G.P. Talwar. 2011. Development of a highly immunogenic recombinant candidate vaccine against human chorionic gonadotropin. *Vaccine* **29:** 2341–2348.

21. Dirnhofer, S., P. Koessler, H. Rogatsch, *et al.* 2000. Selective expressions of trophoblastic hormones by lung carcinoma neuroendocrine tumors exclusively produce human chorionic gonadotropin α-subunit (hCGα). *Hum. Pathol.* **31:** 966–972.

22. Dirnhofer, S., P. Koessler, C. Ensinge, *et al.* 1998. Production of trophoblastic hormones by transitional cell carcinoma of the bladder association to tumor stage and grade. *Hum. Pathol.* **29:** 377–382.

23. Louhimo, J., M. Carpelan-Holmstrom, H. Alfthan, *et al.* 2002. Serum hCGβ, CA 72–4 and CEA are independent prognostic factors in colorectal cancer. *Int. J. Cancer* **101:** 545–548.

24. Syrigos, K. N., I. Fyssas, M.M. Konstandoulakis, *et al.* 1998. Beta human chorionic gonadotropin concertations in serum of patients with pancreatic adenocarcinoma. *Gut* **42:** 88–91.

25. Hedstrom, J., R. Grenman, H. Ramsey, *et al.* 1999. Concentration of free hCGβ subunit in serum as a prognostic marker for squamous-cell carcinoma of the oral cavity and oropharynx. *Int. J. Cancer* **84:** 525–528.

26. Crawford, R.A., R.K. Iles, P.G. Carter, *et al.* 1998. The prognostic significance of human chorionic gonadotropin and its metabolites in women with cervical carcinoma. *J. Clin. Pathol.* **51:** 685–688.

27. Gillott, D.J., R.K. lles & T. Chard. 1996. The effects of b-human chorionic gonadotrophin on the in vitro growth of bladder cancer cell lines. *Br. J. Cancer* **73:** 323–326.

28. Talwar, G.P, J.C. Gupta & N.V. Shankar. 2011. Immunological approaches against human chorionic gonadotrophin for control of fertility and therapy of advanced stage cancers expressing hCG/subunits. *Am. J. Reprod. Immunol.* **66:** 26–39.

29. Kumar, S., G.P. Talwar, & D.K. Biswas. 1992. Necrosis and inhibition of growth of human lung tumor by anti-alpha human chorionic gonadotropin antibody. *J. Natl. Cancer* **84:** 42–47.

30. Vyas, H.K., R. Pal, R. Vishwakarma, *et al.* 2009. Selective killing of leukemia and lymphoma cells ectopically expressing hCG β by a conjugate of curcumin with an antibody against hCGβ subunit. *Oncology* **76:** 101–111.

Ann. N.Y. Acad. Sci. ISSN 0077-8923

Immunology of neuromyelitis optica: a T cell–B cell collaboration

Meike Mitsdoerffer,[1] Vijay Kuchroo,[2] and Thomas Korn[1,3]

[1]Department of Neurology, Klinikum rechts der Isar, Technische Universität München, Munich, Germany. [2]Center for Neurologic Diseases, Brigham and Women's Hospital, Harvard Medical School, Boston, Massachusetts. [3]Munich Cluster for Systems Neurology (SyNergy), Munich, Germany

Address for correspondence: Thomas Korn, Department of Neurology, Klinikum rechts der Isar, Technische Universität München, Ismaninger Str. 22, 81675 Munich, Germany. korn@lrz.tum.de

Neuromyelitis optica (NMO) is a debilitating autoimmune inflammatory disease of the central nervous system (CNS) that is distinct from multiple sclerosis (MS). The discovery of NMO-immunoglobulin G (IgG) in the serum of NMO—but not MS—patients was a breakthrough in defining diagnostic criteria for NMO. NMO-IgG is an antibody directed against the astrocytic water channel protein aquaporin-4 (AQP4). While there is evidence that NMO-IgG is also involved in mediating tissue damage in the CNS, many aspects of the pathogenic cascade in NMO remain to be determined. It is clear that antigen-specific T cells contribute to the generation of NMO-IgG in the peripheral immune compartment, as well as to the development of NMO lesions in the CNS. T helper 17 (Th17) cells, equipped both in providing B cell help and inducing tissue inflammation, may be involved in NMO development and pathogenesis. Here, we review immunologic aspects of NMO, placing recent findings in the biology of T–B cell cooperation into perspective with autoimmunity of the CNS.

Keywords: neuromyelitis optica; inflammation; CNS

Introduction

Neuromyelitis optica (NMO) is an inflammatory demyelinating disease of the central nervous system (CNS) in which lesions occur predominantly in the spinal cord and optic nerves.[1] For several years, it has been a matter of debate as to whether NMO was a distinct disease entity or a variant of multiple sclerosis (MS). Like conventional MS, NMO often shows a relapsing–remitting course.[2] However, NMO is distinct from MS in several aspects, including clinical, neuroimaging, cerebrospinal fluid (CSF), and serological features.[2,3] While patients with MS typically have mild attacks with good recovery, attacks of NMO produce severe disability, often with incomplete recovery. After six years, about one-third of NMO patients have permanent motor disability, one-fourth are wheel chair–bound, one-fifth have bilateral visual disability, and 10% will have died;[4] complications such as respiratory failure have also been reported.[5] However, in contrast to MS, it is uncommon for clinical disability in NMO to progress independently of relapses,[6] suggesting that the pathogenic cascades in NMO and MS are different. Epidemiologic data reveal a pronounced preponderance of women over men afflicted with NMO, compared with MS patients (9:1 vs. 2:1, respectively).[2,7] While brain MRI scans often show no or few inflammatory lesions in NMO patients, longitudinally extensive signal abnormalities can be detected in the spinal cord during acute attacks, typically extending over three or more vertebral segments.[2,7] Analysis of the CSF occasionally reveals a striking pleocytosis, with a polymorph nuclear predominance. Oligoclonal bands of immunoglobulin G (IgG) are observed in a minority of NMO patients (whereas they occur in about 85% of MS patients).[8]

Defining NMO as a distinct disease entity came from the identification of a highly specific serum antibody, NMO-IgG, which is absent in patients with conventional MS.[9] Thus, clinical, imaging, and

doi: 10.1111/nyas.12118

serological hallmarks have led to the conclusion that NMO is a distinct disease entity with specific diagnostic criteria.[3]

Pathologic features of NMO

Historic reports on histopathologic findings in autopsy and biopsy material from patients with NMO highlighted acute spinal cord lesions with diffuse swelling and tissue softening involving several spinal segments and, occasionally, the entire spinal cord in a patchy or continuous distribution.[10, 11] A comparison of lesions in patients who suffered from conventional MS or NMO revealed a unique pathological pattern in the latter: the presence of immunoglobulins located near activated complement in perivascular regions constitutes a prominent feature of NMO lesions.[12] Activated complement (C3a and C5a) has chemoattractant properties that facilitate the recruitment of macrophages and eosinophils into lesion sites. Both eosinophils and macrophages have the ability to mediate complement- and antibody-dependent cytotoxicity via either complement or Ig/Fc receptors, respectively. In addition, activated macrophages, together with eosinophils and neutrophils, can locally generate cytokines, proteases, and either reactive oxygen or nitrogen species, resulting in nonselective bystander destruction of both gray and white matter structures, including axons and oligodendrocytes. Additional characteristics of NMO lesions are increased vascular permeability and edema that might secondarily aggravate tissue destruction via edema-induced ischemia.[13, 14] These observations suggested an important role for humoral immune mechanisms in the pathogenesis of NMO.

The recent identification of a specific serum autoantibody, NMO-IgG, which targets aquaporin-4 (AQP4), the most abundant water channel in the CNS, strengthened the hypothesis of a humoral mechanism in NMO pathogenesis.[9, 15] Interestingly, the distribution pattern of AQP4 expression at glial–fluid interfaces (e.g., perivascular foot processes of astrocytes and at the glia limitans) mirrors the sites of immunoglobulin and complement deposition detected in NMO lesions.[9, 12] In NMO lesions, AQP4 expression is lost, and reduced immunoreactivity to AQP4 correlates with the loss, or reduction, of glial fibrillary acidic protein (GFAP) immunostaining, while myelin basic protein expression is rela-

tively preserved, indicating primary structural damage of astrocytes but not oligodendrocytes. Thus, NMO might principally be an astrocyte disease, with demyelination being a secondary event in lesion development.[16, 17]

While the expression pattern of AQP4 in the CNS and lesion topography in NMO largely support the idea that AQP4 is a target of the immune response in NMO, the correlation of AQP4 expression and lesion topography is not entirely straightforward (see below). Moreover, loss of AQP4 in NMO lesions is associated with structural damage to astrocytes, as indicated by concomitant loss of GFAP immunoreactivity particularly in the spinal cord and optic nerve;[12, 16–18] however, in some niches, NMO lesions appear to be nondestructive. For example, NMO lesions in the area postrema at the floor of the fourth ventricle are characterized by loss of AQP4, with preserved GFAP expression in astrocytes.[19] The reason for the nondestructive and reversible nature of NMO lesions in the area postrema is unclear, although specific properties of area postrema astrocytes, including expression of complement regulatory proteins and lack of coexpression of the glutamate transporter EAAT2 (Glt-1) with AQP4 have been speculated to contribute to their resistance to NMO-IgG–mediated destruction.[19] In contrast to NMO lesions, in which loss of AQP4 immunoreactivity is a unifying feature, AQP4 appears to be upregulated in the periplaque white matter of early- and late-active MS lesions. Only long-standing inactive lesions are characterized by a reduced immunoreactivity for AQP4, while remyelinating lesions (shadow plaques) show a diffusely increased expression of AQP4. Together, the expression of AQP4 follows a stage-dependent pattern correlating with the presence of reactive astrocytes, suggesting that—as opposed to NMO—AQP4 is not the primary target of the immunopathologic process in MS.[16, 17] Another interesting difference between NMO and MS is the degree of cortical demyelination, which is well documented in MS but appears to be absent in NMO, in spite of cortical astrogliosis and neuronal pathology.[20, 21] It is unclear whether cortical demyelination is the histopathologic correlate of secondary progression in the clinical course of MS. Yet, this idea would fit well with the observation that secondary progression does not frequently occur in NMO.

Role of NMO-IgG

Tanycytes (the cells lining the third ventricle) and astrocytes express high levels of AQP4, while oligodendrocytes lack expression of this water channel. AQP4 plays an important, yet probably redundant, role in water homeostasis at the blood–brain and CSF–brain barriers.[22] Indeed, AQP4 knockout mice do not show a spontaneous phenotype.[23] Both AQP4 and AQP1 mediate water flux and seem to be involved in the development of brain edema in pathologic conditions.[24–27] About 70% of all NMO patients have antibodies to AQP4,[28] the majority of which recognize an extracellular determinant in the C-loop of AQP4. NMO-IgG is mainly of the IgG1 subclass and therefore capable of activating complement.[29]

Several clinical and histopathologic lines of evidence support the idea that NMO-IgG has a direct role in disease development. First, therapeutic plasmapheresis is an effective treatment for NMO patients.[30–32] Second, AQP4 antibody titers seem to correlate with clinical severity of the disease.[33–35] Third, regions of the brain and spinal cord that express AQP4 are preferential lesion sites in NMO;[16,17,36] for example, AQP4 is abundantly expressed in the gray matter of the spinal cord, and the periventricular and periaqueductal areas,[37,38] which are also the predominant locations of NMO lesions. Fourth, complement deposition and inflammatory infiltrates of eosinophils can be found in areas of the CNS where astrocytes highly express AQP4, suggesting that NMO-IgG supports the effector functions of complement binding and C1 activation, as well as cell-mediated cytotoxicity, both of which lead to structural damage of astrocytes[16,17,39] (Fig. 1). It remains controversial whether binding of NMO-IgG also leads to functional alterations of AQP4, for example disturbed water and solute homeostasis, or internalization of AQP4, with formation of cytotoxic edema as a potential consequence.[40,41]

Recent studies have investigated potential effector functions of NMO-IgG in greater detail. AQP4 antibody and complement factors have been shown to induce necrosis of astrocytes *in vitro*.[42] In addition, from coculture systems of astrocytes and oligodendrocytes it was proposed that NMO-IgG might bind to astrocytes and disturb glutamate homeostasis; in support of this, downregulation of EAAT2 in astrocytes has been shown to result in impaired

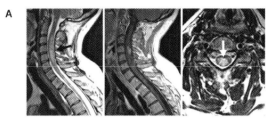

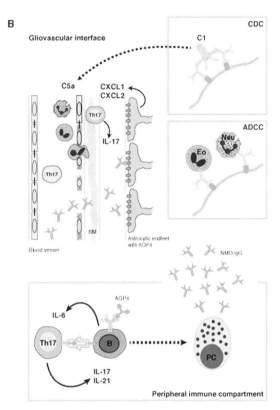

Figure 1. Longitudinal extensive transverse myelitis is a defining feature of NMO. (A) In the left panel: T2w image of the cervicothoracic spinal cord of a patient with NMO. Note the extension of the centromedullary lesion (arrow) over more than three vertebral segments. Middle panel: Contrast-enhanced T1w image of the same lesion. Right panel: T2w image (transverse section) showing the centromedullary location of the NMO lesion (arrow). (B) Pathogenic process in NMO: in the peripheral immune compartment, B cells bearing an AQP4-specific B cell receptor might serve as antigen-presenting cells to prime autoreactive T cells to develop into the Th17 lineage. In turn, Th17 cells have the ability to help B cells become plasma cells, producing antibodies to AQP4 (NMO-IgG). These serum antibodies that are not per se produced intrathecally only cross the blood–brain barrier, including the endothelial basement membrane (BM) under conditions of ongoing inflammation of the endothelium of the CNS vasculature, which might again be driven by Th17 cells. Upon binding of their target antigen (i.e., AQP4 expressed

Continued

glutamate uptake into astrocytes and cause glutamate excitotoxicity in neighboring oligodendrocytes, and demyelination in *ex vivo* experiments.[18,43] However, appropriate animal models of NMO are still needed to test these hypotheses *in vivo*.

Systemic transfer of NMO-IgG alone into experimental animals did not provoke disease activity. This might be due, in part, to limited ability of serum proteins to pass the blood–brain or blood–CSF barriers into the CNS compartment. On the other hand, lack of a tight blood–brain barrier appears not to be sufficient for NMO-IgG to exert its effector functions in the CNS, as NMO-IgG transfer into juvenile laboratory animals, which have a leaky blood–brain barrier, fail to induce pathology.[44]

In fact, the necessary component for induction of NMO-IgG–mediated pathology is inflammatory alterations of the blood–brain barrier. Most likely, AQP4 antibodies only become pathogenic at sites of inflammation in the presence of either activated effector cells or sufficient amounts of complement in the absence of complement inhibitory factors. Passive transfer of NMO-IgG into experimental autoimmune encephalomyelitis (EAE) rats—which had been immunized to develop a subclinical T cell response against a myelin antigen—not only exacerbated EAE severity but also caused striking histopathologic changes reminiscent of NMO lesions, including extensive loss of astrocytes as well as perivascular deposition of immunoglobulin and complement.[44–46] Loss of AQP4 extended beyond the borders of the structurally damaged area, and some areas adjacent to the lesions showed astrocytic processes devoid of AQP4 but with preserved GFAP expression.[44] Interestingly, a recent study showed that coinjection of NMO-IgG and human complement directly into the cerebrum of experimental mice was sufficient to provoke NMO-like lesions, with loss of AQP4 expression and glial cell edema.[47] These data indicate that T cells might be dispensable for the effector functions of NMO-IgG at the lesion site, albeit under experimental conditions

in which the blood–brain barrier has been short-circuited and when a permissive (i.e., inflammatory and complement-sufficient) milieu is created by the approach.[47] However, NMO-IgG alone, even after trafficking into the CNS, may not be sufficient to induce NMO lesions. Circumventricular organs, such as the area postrema, lack a tight blood–brain barrier even under physiological (i.e., noninflammatory) conditions, and it is in these areas, not in other sites of the CNS, that binding of intravenously injected NMO-IgG can be detected but does not induce structural damage.[48]

Therefore, whereas NMO-IgG specific for AQP4 is pathognomonic for NMO, the presence of T cells, complement, and inflammation is required for the development of parenchymal tissue damage in NMO. Hence, there are still uncertainties regarding the exact effector mechanisms and the overall impact of anti-AQP4 antibodies. Although the topography of NMO lesions has been associated with the distribution of AQP4 expression in the CNS,[8,38] it is incompletely understood why certain areas of the CNS, including the cortical gray matter, appear to be preserved from NMO lesions despite an abundance of AQP4 expression in cortical astrocytes. In addition, AQP4 is highly expressed in peripheral tissues, including gastric mucosa, kidney, and muscle; yet, seropositive NMO patients do not suffer from clinically apparent interstitial nephritis or myositis. One explanation might be that the AQP4 clustering in orthogonal arrays of particles leads to the generation of pathogenic epitopes only at particular sites of the CNS.[49] The M23 isoform of AQP4 forms orthogonal arrays of particles and may react differentially to NMO-IgG binding, compared with the M1 isoform. Another hypothesis is that the absence of complement inhibitory or regulatory factors might favor NMO-IgG–mediated pathology only in certain anatomical niches.[50]

T cell specificity in NMO

Since the discovery of NMO-IgG in 2004, NMO has been regarded primarily as an antibody-mediated disease. However, a series of studies have provided evidence for an important role for effector T cells in various steps of NMO pathogenesis.[44] As mentioned above, the presence of AQP4-specific antibodies alone is not sufficient to provoke inflammatory disease in the CNS; indeed, some patients show persistently high titers of anti-AQP4

---

in astrocytic endfeet of the glia limitans), NMO-IgG initiate a downstream pathogenic cascade leading to tissue damage either by complement-dependent cytotoxicity (CDC, upper box) or antibody-dependent cell-mediated cytotoxicity (ADCC, lower box). Here, eosinophils (Eo) recruited into the lesion by C5a, or neutrophils (Neu) recruited into the lesion by ELR chemokines such as CXCL1 and CXCL2, are potential effector cells.

antibodies despite clinical remission.[51–54] Transfer of *in vitro*–generated, AQP4 peptide-specific T cells into rats in the absence of NMO-IgG was shown to provoke a subclinical disease, with inflammatory lesions along the entire neuroaxis. In contrast, cotransfer of AQP4-specific T cells plus NMO-IgG resulted in inflammatory tissue damage reminiscent of NMO.[55] Thus, effector T cells seem to be required for lesion development, at least for disrupting the blood–brain or blood–CSF barriers, and perhaps for creating an inflammatory milieu *in situ* for antibodies to be operational. T cells are also found within the lesions of NMO patients, though their antigen specificity and function have not been characterized.

In a different sense, it is clear that AQP4-specific T cells are required in the peripheral immune compartment to help B cells generate production of NMO-IgG, a class-switched antibody (Fig. 1). Some efforts have been made to define AQP4-specific T cells in NMO patients. However, the AQP4 epitopes restricted to HLA alleles that are overrepresented in NMO patients (e.g., DR17 (DRB1*0301)) have not been identified.[56,57] T cells from NMO patients have been shown to respond to an immunodominant DR-restricted AQP4 epitope (AA61–80),[58] although the exact haplotype restriction was not determined. Interestingly, a study on 11 Japanese NMO patients showed a clonal expansion of T cells expressing $V_\beta 1$ and $V_\beta 13$ chains,[59] although no information was given on the patients' HLA status; in Japanese cohorts, HLA-DPB1*0501, but not DRB1*0301, is overrepresented in anti-AQP4 antibody positive NMO patients.[53] Recent studies in mice identified the major immunogenic T cell epitopes of AQP4 presented by I-A^b.[60,61] Thus, it might be possible to build experimental models that allow investigation of anti-AQP4–specific adaptive immune responses similar to myelin oligodendrocyte glycoprotein (MOG)–specific responses, but utilizing the putatively correct autoantigen AQP4 implicated in the development of NMO. It would then be possible to ask questions about the cytokine phenotype, the timing, and the relevant compartments of adaptive immune responses against AQP4.

T cell phenotype in NMO

Upon antigen-specific activation, T helper cells become effector T cells that produce cytokines. T helper cells have been classified into various subsets on the basis of specific signature effector cytokines with distinct functions.[62] The different subsets, or T helper cell lineages, are distinguished from one another on the basis of the differentiation factors (usually produced by innate immune cells or antigen-presenting cells like B cells) required to begin a specific developmental program leading to activated T helper cell subtypes; the individual developmental programs require distinct transcriptional modules controlled by specific transcription factors. For example, innate immune cell-derived interleukin (IL)-12 is necessary for the development of Th1 cells, which express the transcription factor T-bet and produce interferon (IFN)-γ as a signature cytokine; Th2 cells are induced by IL-4, express Gata3, and produce IL-4, IL-5, and IL-13. Th17 cells are induced by a combination of TGF-β plus IL-6, with IL-21 and IL-23 enhancing their precursor frequency and stabilizing their phenotype, respectively; Th17 cells express the transcription factor RORγt and produce IL-17, IL-21, and IL-22.[63,64] The various T helper cell lineages have specific functions in host defense. While Th1 cells are required to control viruses and intracellular bacteria, Th2 cells orchestrate the immune response against parasites; Th17 cells are important for immune responses to certain extracellular bacteria and fungi.

Immunopathology in organ-specific autoimmunity—such as that in MS—is believed to be due to dysregulated Th1 and Th17 responses, as Th1 and Th17 cells and their effector molecule signatures are found in the CSF and in MS lesions.[65] However, secondary inflammatory infiltrates in MS are dominated by macrophages, which are activated by IFN-γ, while neutrophils, which are attracted by IL-17–induced chemokines, are rare in MS lesions and absent in the CSF of MS patients.[66] Compared with MS patients, NMO patients have elevated IL-6 and IL-17 in the CSF;[67,68] and consistent with this, NMO patients display higher proportions of Th17 cells and IL-17–producing CD8$^+$ T cells in the peripheral blood, compared with controls.[58,69] Thus, it is possible that NMO is actually a paradigm for a Th17-driven autoimmune disease.[70]

However, if NMO is a Th17-mediated autoimmune disease, how can this be reconciled with the prominent role of B cells in NMO, including potential effector functions of NMO-IgG? In fact, there is increasing evidence of extensive cross talk (in both directions) between Th17 and B cells. And while the cellular sources of IL-6 and IL-23 for the differentiation of Th17 cells have not been defined *in vivo*, it is possible that B cells, which can serve as antigen-presenting cells in the context of NMO and are an excellent source of IL-6, might skew T cells toward a Th17 response (Fig. 1). Also, it has been demonstrated that Th17 cells provide very effective help to B cells.[71] Consistent with this idea, the presence of high frequencies of Th17 cells was shown to be sufficient to drive the generation of germinal centers and the production of autoantibodies (anti-GPI) to induce arthritis in K/BxN mice.[72] Furthermore, MOG-specific Th17 cells have been shown to have the unique ability to induce the generation of ectopic lymphoid follicles in the subarachnoid space upon transfer into naive recipient mice; this was partly dependent on the expression of the cell surface molecule podoplanin and the secretion of IL-17 by MOG-specific Th17 cells.[73]

Detailed analyses of the interaction between T and B cells reactive against the same cognate antigen have been performed in MOG-specific models of CNS autoimmunity. Double-transgenic mice with both T and B cells specific for MOG developed very severe, spontaneous CNS autoimmunity, while the presence of antigen-specific B or T cells alone provoke little or no disease.[74,75] Histopathologic analyses identified the spinal cord and optic nerves as major locations for lesion development in the double-transgenic animals, whereas the brain was devoid of any lesions. Indeed, spontaneous CNS autoimmunity in double-transgenic mice has some of the features of NMO and was proposed to be a model for opticospinal MS. However, comparisons with NMO should be made cautiously since AQP4–but not MOG–may be the relevant autoantigen in NMO. On the other hand, about 30% of NMO patients, diagnosed according to the 2006 criteria,[3] are seronegative for NMO-IgG.[76] Interestingly, the clinical phenotype of the classic Devic's syndrome (i.e., a sequence of monophasic, longitudinal, extensive transverse myelitis and optic neuritis[1]) is quite frequent among seronegative NMO patients, and it has recently been reported that a fraction (16%) of seronegative NMO patients harbor serum antibodies to MOG, which are not found in conventional adult MS patients.[77] Another histopathologic hallmark of EAE in MOG T and B cell receptor double-transgenic mice is the presence of lymph follicle–like structures in the meninges,[74] which

indicate germinal center reactions within the meningeal compartment. In addition, these models suggest that antigen-specific T cells also recruit antigen-specific B cells from the natural repertoire to develop into antibody-producing cells within the subarachnoid and CNS compartments, and thus contribute to lesion development by means of MOG-specific antibodies.[78]

Although these transgenic model systems reflect important histopathologic features of MS, it has been unclear whether the cooperation between MOG-specific T and B cells translates to the case of AQP4 being the disease-relevant target autoantigen. Importantly, in seropositive NMO patients, NMO-IgG is not produced intrathecally (i.e., antibody-producing plasmablasts or plasma cells are not recruited to the subarachnoid space);[79] consistent with this, follicle-like structures in the meninges have not been reported in NMO patients. Rather, it appears that the humoral immune response against AQP4 is exclusively generated in the peripheral immune compartment; this is different from MS. Specifically, intrathecal synthesis of antibodies is frequently observed in MS, with the presence of lymph follicle–like structures in the meninges in about 40%–50% of secondary progressive patients—and was associated with cortical demyelination (which is not found in NMO).

Hence, the contribution of T cells in the pathogenic cascades of MS and NMO appears to be fundamentally different, and much work remains to be done on the actual T cell contribution to the disease process in NMO-IgG seropositive NMO patients, although accumulating data suggest that T cells may have an important role not only in helping B cells but also in collaborating with antibodies in mediating tissue damage.

Therapy of NMO

Treatment regimens for NMO will probably never reach evidence level I (randomized controlled trial; meta-analysis) or even level II (non-randomized clinical trial) simply due to the rarity of NMO: being 100 times less frequent than MS (thus, patient numbers required to test treatment options in randomized trials with adequate power will not be feasible). Yet, since the pathogenic concepts in NMO are quite advanced, therapeutic strategies may be introduced based on these disease mechanisms.

Currently, the standard of care includes treatment of acute attacks, on the one hand, and prophylactic strategies to prevent future attacks, on the other. Intravenous corticosteroid therapy is usually the initial treatment for acute attacks of optic neuritis or myelitis in NMO patients. However, patients who do not respond promptly to corticosteroid treatment might benefit from plasmapheresis, which is recommended to be initiated early, particularly for patients with severe myelitis who are at high risk for neurogenic respiratory failure.[80] While this strategy is broadly accepted for the treatment of attacks, there is some controversy in its use as a prophylactic treatment. In line with the concept that antibodies contribute to the disease mechanism in NMO, treatment of patients with the B cell–depleting anti-CD20 monoclonal antibody rituximab appears to dampen disease activity and prevent relapses.[81,82] Because reappearance of memory B cells after depletion of B cells with anti-CD20 has been observed to be a potential marker of resuming disease activity,[83] efforts are being undertaken to target memory B cells even more efficiently by using a depleting antibody to CD19. In addition, general immunosuppressant agents, such as azathioprine or mycophenolate mofetil, have been used, with mixed responses.[84,85] Novel and more targeted therapies are required for both acute intervention in NMO attacks and long-term immune prophylaxis.

The knowledge of potential effector functions of NMO-IgG has been used to design new targeted therapeutic approaches. For example, a recombinant anti-AQP4 antibody has been developed that binds to the C-loop of AQP4 but lacks the effector functions of NMO-IgG (i.e., it does not lead to complement fixation and antibody-dependent cell-mediated cytotoxicity that is eosinophil mediated; Fig. 1). This recombinant antibody, aquaporumab, is thought to competitively bind the AQP4 epitope and prevent pathogenic NMO-IgG from binding; it has been shown to block cell surface AQP4 binding of polyclonal NMO-IgG derived from NMO patient sera in cell culture and in *ex vivo* spinal cord slices, as well as in an *in vivo* mouse model. As a consequence of AQP4 epitope occupancy by aquaporumab (or other small molecule inhibitors), downstream cytotoxicity of NMO-IgG and formation of typical NMO lesions was suppressed.[86,87] Another therapeutic strategy to treat NMO relapses made use of eculizumab, a monoclonal antibody against C5, which inhibits its cleavage by the C5 convertase and, thus, prevents complement activation.

In summary, information on NMO pathogenesis has been promptly translated into clinical treatment strategies for NMO attacks. However, regarding immune prophylactic therapies, the standard of care in NMO still largely relies on nonselective immunosuppression to inhibit the generation of NMO-IgG in the peripheral immune compartment. Unfortunately, some immune prophylactic therapies, including interferons, fingolimod, and natalizumab, which are beneficial in MS, have been shown to be ineffective when used in individual NMO patients or in NMO patient series.[88–93] It might be useful to target molecules related to the biology of Th17 cells, as anti–IL-17 treatment appears to be safe and works very well in other Th17-related diseases, such as psoriasis.[94] A monoclonal antibody to the IL-6 receptor (tocilizumab) was proven effective in severe cases of NMO that were refractory to standard of care treatment.[95,96]

It will be a major challenge in future research to improve, and then apply, the knowledge on antigen-specific adaptive immune responses against AQP4 to design well-tolerated, antigen- or phenotype-specific, immune prophylactic therapies to prevent debilitating NMO relapses in the first place.

Acknowledgments

We thank Dr. Claus Zimmer (Department of Neuroradiology, Klinikum rechts der Isar) for providing the MRI images. This work was supported by intramural funding (KKF) to M.M. (B02–12). V.K.K. is supported by the Guthy-Jackson Charitable Foundation and by grants from the NIH. T.K. is recipient of a Heisenberg Award from the DFG (KO2964/3–2). This work was supported by the DFG (SFB TR 128/A06 and grants within the framework of the Munich Cluster for Systems Neurology (EXC 1010 SyNergy)).

Conflicts of interest

The authors declare no conflicts of interest.

References

1. Devic, E. 1894. Myélite subaiguë compliquée de névrite optique. *Bull Med (Paris).* **8:** 1033–1034.
2. Wingerchuk, D.M. *et al.* 1999. The clinical course of neuromyelitis optica (Devic's syndrome). *Neurology* **53:** 1107–1114.

3. Wingerchuk, D.M. *et al.* 2006. Revised diagnostic criteria for neuromyelitis optica. *Neurology* **66:** 1485–1489.

4. Kitley, J. *et al.* 2012. Prognostic factors and disease course in aquaporin-4 antibody-positive patients with neuromyelitis optica spectrum disorder from the United Kingdom and Japan. *Brain* **135:** 1834–1849.

5. Kobayashi, Z. *et al.* 2009. Intractable hiccup caused by medulla oblongata lesions: a study of an autopsy patient with possible neuromyelitis optica. *J. Neurol. Sci.* **285:** 241–245.

6. Wingerchuk, D.M. *et al.* 2007. A secondary progressive clinical course is uncommon in neuromyelitis optica. *Neurology* **68:** 603–605.

7. O'Riordan, J.I. *et al.* 1996. Clinical, CSF, and MRI findings in Devic's neuromyelitis optica. *J. Neurol. Neurosurg. Psychiatry* **60:** 382–387.

8. Wingerchuk, D.M. *et al.* 2007. The spectrum of neuromyelitis optica. *Lancet Neurol.* **6:** 805–815.

9. Lennon, V.A. *et al.* 2004. A serum autoantibody marker of neuromyelitis optica: distinction from multiple sclerosis. *Lancet* **364:** 2106–2112.

10. Cloys, D.E. & M.G. Netsky. 1970. *Neuromyelitis Optica.* Amsterdam: North Holland Publishing Co.

11. Mandler, R.N. *et al.* 1993. Devic's neuromyelitis optica: a clinicopathological study of 8 patients. *Ann Neurol.* **34:** 162–168.

12. Lucchinetti, C.F. *et al.* 2002. A role for humoral mechanisms in the pathogenesis of Devic's neuromyelitis optica. *Brain* **125:** 1450–1461.

13. Prineas, J.W. & W.I. McDonald. 1997. Demyelinating diseases. In Graham, D. I. Lantos, P. L. (eds.): *Greenfield's Neuropathology*, 6th edition, Arnold, London, pp. 813–896.

14. Aboul-Enein, F. *et al.* 2003. Preferential loss of myelin-associated glycoprotein reflects hypoxia-like white matter damage in stroke and inflammatory brain diseases. *J. Neuropathol. Exp. Neurol.* **62:** 25–33.

15. Lennon, V.A. *et al.* 2005. IgG marker of optic-spinal multiple sclerosis binds to the aquaporin-4 water channel. *J. Exp. Med.* **202:** 473–477.

16. Misu, T. *et al.* 2007. Loss of aquaporin 4 in lesions of neuromyelitis optica: distinction from multiple sclerosis. *Brain* **130:** 1224–1234.

17. Roemer, S.F. *et al.* 2007. Pattern-specific loss of aquaporin-4 immunoreactivity distinguishes neuromyelitis optica from multiple sclerosis. *Brain* **130:** 1194–1205.

18. Hinson, S.R. *et al.* 2008. Aquaporin-4-binding autoantibodies in patients with neuromyelitis optica impair glutamate transport by down-regulating EAAT2. *J. Exp. Med.* **205:** 2473–2481.

19. Popescu, B.F. *et al.* 2011. Neuromyelitis optica unique area postrema lesions: nausea, vomiting, and pathogenic implications. *Neurology* **76:** 1229–1237.

20. Lucchinetti, C.F. *et al.* 2011. Inflammatory cortical demyelination in early multiple sclerosis. *N. Eng. J. Med.* **365:** 2188–2197.

21. Popescu, B.F. *et al.* 2010. Absence of cortical demyelination in neuromyelitis optica. *Neurology* **75:** 2103–2109.

22. Nicchia, G.P. *et al.* 2004. The role of aquaporin-4 in the blood-brain barrier development and integrity: studies in animal and cell culture models. *Neuroscience* **129:** 935–945.

23. Ma, T. *et al.* 1997. Generation and phenotype of a transgenic knockout mouse lacking the mercurial-insensitive water channel aquaporin-4. *J. Clin. Invest.* **100:** 957–962.

24. Manley, G.T. *et al.* 2000. Aquaporin-4 deletion in mice reduces brain edema after acute water intoxication and ischemic stroke. *Nat. Med.* **6:** 159–163.

25. Saadoun, S. *et al.* 2002. Aquaporin-4 expression is increased in oedematous human brain tumours. *J. Neurol. Neurosurg. Psychiatry* **72:** 262–265.

26. Taniguchi, M. *et al.* 2000. Induction of aquaporin-4 water channel mRNA after focal cerebral ischemia in rat. *Brain Res. Mol. Brain Res.* **78:** 131–137.

27. Warth, A., M. Mittelbronn & H. Wolburg. 2005. Redistribution of the water channel protein aquaporin-4 and the K$^+$ channel protein Kir4.1 differs in low- and high-grade human brain tumors. *Acta Neuropathol.* **109:** 418–426.

28. Waters, P. *et al.* 2008. Aquaporin-4 antibodies in neuromyelitis optica and longitudinally extensive transverse myelitis. *Arch Neurol.* **65:** 913–919.

29. Hinson, S.R. *et al.* 2007. Pathogenic potential of IgG binding to water channel extracellular domain in neuromyelitis optica. *Neurology* **69:** 2221–2231.

30. Jarius, S. *et al.* 2008. Mechanisms of disease: aquaporin-4 antibodies in neuromyelitis optica. *Nat. Clin. Pract. Neurol.* **4:** 202–214.

31. Matiello, M. *et al.* 2007. Neuromyelitis optica. *Curr. Opin. Neurol.* **20:** 255–260.

32. Watanabe, S. *et al.* 2007. Therapeutic efficacy of plasma exchange in NMO-IgG-positive patients with neuromyelitis optica. *Mult. Scler.* **13:** 128–132.

33. Jarius, S. *et al.* 2008. Antibody to aquaporin-4 in the long-term course of neuromyelitis optica. *Brain* **131:** 3072–3080.

34. Takahashi, T. *et al.* 2007. Anti-aquaporin-4 antibody is involved in the pathogenesis of NMO: a study on antibody titre. *Brain* **130:** 1235–1243.

35. Weinstock-Guttman, B. *et al.* 2008. Neuromyelitis optica immunoglobulins as a marker of disease activity and response to therapy in patients with neuromyelitis optica. *Mult. Scler.* **14:** 1061–1067.

36. Pittock, S.J. *et al.* 2006. Neuromyelitis optica brain lesions localized at sites of high aquaporin 4 expression. *Arch. Neurol.* **63:** 964–968.

37. Oshio, K. *et al.* 2004. Expression of aquaporin water channels in mouse spinal cord. *Neuroscience* **127:** 685–693.

38. Saini, H. *et al.* 2010. Differential expression of aquaporin-4 isoforms localizes with neuromyelitis optica disease activity. *J. Neuroimmunol.* **221:** 68–72.

39. Matsuoka, T. *et al.* 2007. Heterogeneity of aquaporin-4 autoimmunity and spinal cord lesions in multiple sclerosis in Japanese. *Brain* **130:** 1206–1223.

40. Hinson, S.R. *et al.* 2012. Molecular outcomes of neuromyelitis optica (NMO)-IgG binding to aquaporin-4 in astrocytes. *Proc. Natl. Acad. Sci. USA* **109:** 1245–1250.

41. Ratelade, J., J.L. Bennett & A.S. Verkman. 2011. Evidence against cellular internalization in vivo of NMO-IgG, aquaporin-4, and excitatory amino acid transporter 2 in neuromyelitis optica. *J. Biol. Chem.* **286:** 45156–45164.

42. Kinoshita, M. *et al.* 2009. Astrocytic necrosis is induced by anti-aquaporin-4 antibody-positive serum. *Neuroreport* **20:** 508–512.

43. Marignier, R. *et al.* 2010. Oligodendrocytes are damaged by neuromyelitis optica immunoglobulin G via astrocyte injury. *Brain* **133:** 2578–2591.

44. Bradl, M. *et al.* 2009. Neuromyelitis optica: pathogenicity of patient immunoglobulin in vivo. *Ann. Neurol.* **66:** 630–643.

45. Bennett, J.L. *et al.* 2009. Intrathecal pathogenic anti-aquaporin-4 antibodies in early neuromyelitis optica. *Ann. Neurol.* **66:** 617–629.

46. Kinoshita, M. *et al.* 2009. Neuromyelitis optica: passive transfer to rats by human immunoglobulin. *Biochem. Biophys. Res. Commun.* **386:** 623–627.

47. Saadoun, S. *et al.* 2010. Intra-cerebral injection of neuromyelitis optica immunoglobulin G and human complement produces neuromyelitis optica lesions in mice. *Brain* **133:** 349–361.

48. Ratelade, J., J.L. Bennett & A.S. Verkman. 2011. Intravenous neuromyelitis optica autoantibody in mice targets aquaporin-4 in peripheral organs and area postrema. *PLoS One* **6:** e27412.

49. Nicchia, G.P. *et al.* 2008. Expression of multiple AQP4 pools in the plasma membrane and their association with the dystrophin complex. *J. Neurochem.* **105:** 2156–2165.

50. Zipfel, P.F. & C. Skerka. 2009. Complement regulators and inhibitory proteins. *Nat. Rev. Immunol.* **9:** 729–740.

51. Nishiyama, S. *et al.* 2009. A case of NMO seropositive for aquaporin-4 antibody more than 10 years before onset. *Neurology* **72:** 1960–1961.

52. Pittock, S.J. *et al.* 2008. Neuromyelitis optica and non organ-specific autoimmunity. *Arch. Neurol.* **65:** 78–83.

53. Matsushita, T. *et al.* 2009. Association of the HLA-DPB1*0501 allele with anti-aquaporin-4 antibody positivity in Japanese patients with idiopathic central nervous system demyelinating disorders. *Tissue Antigens* **73:** 171–176.

54. Leite, M.I. *et al.* 2012. Myasthenia gravis and neuromyelitis optica spectrum disorder: a multicenter study of 16 patients. *Neurology* **78:** 1601–1607.

55. Pohl, M. *et al.* 2011. Pathogenic T cell responses against aquaporin 4. *Acta Neuropathol. (Berl.)* **122:** 21–34.

56. Brum, D.G. *et al.* 2010. HLA-DRB association in neuromyelitis optica is different from that observed in multiple sclerosis. *Mult. Scler.* **16:** 21–29.

57. Deschamps, R. *et al.* 2011. Different HLA class II (DRB1 and DQB1) alleles determine either susceptibility or resistance to NMO and multiple sclerosis among the French Afro-Caribbean population. *Mult. Scler.* **17:** 24–31.

58. Varrin-Doyer, M. *et al.* 2012. Aquaporin 4-specific T cells in neuromyelitis optica exhibit a Th17 bias and recognize Clostridium ABC transporter. *Ann. Neurol.* **72:** 53–64.

59. Warabi, Y. *et al.* 2006. Characterization of the T cell receptor repertoire in the Japanese neuromyelitis optica: T cell activity is up-regulated compared to multiple sclerosis. *J. Neurol. Sci.* **249:** 145–152.

60. Kalluri, S.R. *et al.* 2011. Functional characterization of aquaporin-4 specific T cells: towards a model for neuromyelitis optica. *PLoS One* **6:** e16083.

61. Nelson, P.A. *et al.* 2010. Immunodominant T cell determinants of aquaporin-4, the autoantigen associated with neuromyelitis optica. *PLoS One* **5:** e15050.

62. Mosmann, T.R. & R.L. Coffman. 1989. TH1 and TH2 cells: different patterns of lymphokine secretion lead to different functional properties. *Annu. Rev. Immunol.* **7:** 145–173.

63. Murphy, K.M. & S.L. Reiner. 2002. The lineage decisions of helper T cells. *Nat. Rev. Immunol.* **2:** 933–944.

64. Korn, T. *et al.* 2009. IL-17 and Th17 cells. *Annu. Rev. Immunol.* **27:** 485–517.

65. Korn, T., M. Mitsdoerffer & V.K. Kuchroo. 2010. Immunological basis for the development of tissue inflammation and organ-specific autoimmunity in animal models of multiple sclerosis. *Results Probl. Cell Differ.* **51:** 43–74.

66. Sospedra, M. & R. Martin. 2005. Immunology of multiple sclerosis. *Annu. Rev. Immunol.* **23:** 683–747.

67. Ishizu, T. *et al.* 2005. Intrathecal activation of the IL-17/IL-8 axis in opticospinal multiple sclerosis. *Brain* **128:** 988–1002.

68. Uzawa, A. *et al.* 2009. Markedly increased CSF interleukin-6 levels in neuromyelitis optica, but not in multiple sclerosis. *J. Neurol.* **256:** 2082–2084.

69. Wang, H.H. *et al.* 2011. Interleukin-17-secreting T cells in neuromyelitis optica and multiple sclerosis during relapse. *J. Clin. Neurosci.* **18:** 1313–1317.

70. Kira, J. 2011. Neuromyelitis optica and opticospinal multiple sclerosis: mechanisms and pathogenesis. *Pathophysiology* **18:** 69–79.

71. Mitsdoerffer, M. *et al.* 2010. Proinflammatory T helper type 17 cells are effective B-cell helpers. *Proc. Natl. Acad. Sci. USA* **107:** 14292–14297.

72. Wu, H.J. *et al.* 2010. Gut-residing segmented filamentous bacteria drive autoimmune arthritis via T helper 17 cells. *Immunity* **32:** 815–827.

73. Peters, A. *et al.* 2011. Th17 cells induce ectopic lymphoid follicles in central nervous system tissue inflammation. *Immunity* **35:** 986–996.

74. Bettelli, E. *et al.* 2006. Myelin oligodendrocyte glycoprotein-specific T and B cells cooperate to induce a Devic-like disease in mice. *J. Clin. Invest.* **116:** 2393–2402.

75. Krishnamoorthy, G. *et al.* 2006. Spontaneous opticospinal encephalomyelitis in a double-transgenic mouse model of autoimmune T cell/B cell cooperation. *J. Clin. Invest.* **116:** 2385–2392.

76. Mealy, M.A. *et al.* 2012. Epidemiology of neuromyelitis optica in the United States: a multicenter analysis. *Arch. Neurol.* **69:** 1176–1180.

77. Kitley, J. *et al.* 2012. Myelin-oligodendrocyte glycoprotein antibodies in adults with a neuromyelitis optica phenotype. *Neurology* **79:** 1273–1277.

78. Pollinger, B. *et al.* 2009. Spontaneous relapsing-remitting EAE in the SJL/J mouse: MOG-reactive transgenic T cells recruit endogenous MOG-specific B cells. *J. Exp. Med.* **206:** 1303–1316.

79. Kalluri, S.R. *et al.* 2010. Quantification and functional characterization of antibodies to native aquaporin 4 in neuromyelitis optica. *Arch. Neurol.* **67:** 1201–1208.

80. Keegan, M. *et al.* 2002. Plasma exchange for severe attacks of CNS demyelination: predictors of response. *Neurology* **58:** 143–146.

81. Cree, B.A. *et al.* 2005. An open label study of the effects of rituximab in neuromyelitis optica. *Neurology* **64:** 1270–1272.

82. Jacob, A. *et al.* 2008. Treatment of neuromyelitis optica with rituximab: retrospective analysis of 25 patients. *Arch. Neurol.* **65:** 1443–1448.

83. Kim, S.H. *et al.* 2011. Repeated treatment with rituximab based on the assessment of peripheral circulating memory B cells in patients with relapsing neuromyelitis optica over 2 years. *Arch. Neurol.* **68:** 1412–1420.

84. Bichuetti, D.B. *et al.* 2010. Neuromyelitis optica treatment: analysis of 36 patients. *Arch. Neurol.* **67:** 1131–1136.

85. Jacob, A. *et al.* 2009. Treatment of neuromyelitis optica with mycophenolate mofetil: retrospective analysis of 24 patients. *Arch. Neurol.* **66:** 1128–1133.

86. Tradtrantip, L. *et al.* 2012. Anti-aquaporin-4 monoclonal antibody blocker therapy for neuromyelitis optica. *Ann. Neurol.* **71:** 314–322.

87. Phuan, P.W. *et al.* 2012. A small-molecule screen yields idiotype-specific blockers of neuromyelitis optica immunoglobulin G binding to aquaporin-4. *J. Biol. Chem.* **287:** 36837–36844.

88. Papeix, C. *et al.* 2007. Immunosuppressive therapy is more effective than interferon in neuromyelitis optica. *Mult. Scler.* **13:** 256–259.

89. Uzawa, A. *et al.* 2010. Different responses to interferon beta-1b treatment in patients with neuromyelitis optica and multiple sclerosis. *Eur. J. Neurol.* **17:** 672–676.

90. Tanaka, M., K. Tanaka & M. Komori. 2009. Interferon-beta(1b) treatment in neuromyelitis optica. *Eur. Neurol.* **62:** 167–170.

91. Kim, S.H. *et al.* 2012. Does interferon beta treatment exacerbate neuromyelitis optica spectrum disorder? *Mult. Scler.* **18:** 1480–1483.

92. Min, J.H., B.J. Kim & K.H. Lee. 2012. Development of extensive brain lesions following fingolimod (FTY720) treatment in a patient with neuromyelitis optica spectrum disorder. *Mult. Scler.* **18:** 113–115.

93. Kleiter, I. *et al.* 2012. Failure of natalizumab to prevent relapses in neuromyelitis optica. *Arch. Neurol.* **69:** 239–245.

94. Leonardi, C. *et al.* 2012. Anti-interleukin-17 monoclonal antibody ixekizumab in chronic plaque psoriasis. *N. Engl. J. Med.* **366:** 1190–1199.

95. Ayzenberg, I. *et al.* 2013. Interleukin 6 receptor blockade in patients with neuromyelitis optica nonresponsive to anti-CD20 therapy. *JAMA Neuro.* **70:** 394–397.

96. Kieseier, B.C. *et al.* 2012. Disease amelioration with tocilizumab in a treatment-resistant patient with neuromyelitis optica: implication for cellular immune responses. *Arch. Neurol.* 1–4. DOI: 10.1001/jamaneurol.2013.668. [Epub ahead of print].

Ann. N.Y. Acad. Sci. ISSN 0077-8923

ANNALS OF THE NEW YORK ACADEMY OF SCIENCES

Issue: *Translational Immunology in Asia-Oceania*

Regulation of Toll-like receptor signaling pathways in innate immune responses

Cheng Qian[1] and Xuetao Cao[1,2]

[1]National Key Laboratory of Medical Immunology, and Institute of Immunology, Second Military Medical University, Shanghai, China. [2]National Key Laboratory of Medical Molecular Biology, and Department of Immunology, Chinese Academy of Medical Sciences, Beijing, China

Address for correspondence: Dr. Cheng Qian, National Key Laboratory of Medical Immunology & Institute of Immunology, Second Military Medical University, Shanghai 200433, China. crystalqiancheng@yahoo.com.cn; and Dr. Xuetao Cao, National Key Laboratory of Medical Molecular Biology, and Department of Immunology, Chinese Academy of Medical Sciences, Beijing, China. caoxt@immunol.org

Toll-like receptors (TLRs) are critical pattern recognition receptors (PRRs) that recognize pathogen-associated molecular patterns (PAMPs), which are conserved and specific molecular "signatures" expressed by pathogens. TLR ligation triggers distinct but shared signaling pathways that lead to effector mechanisms in innate immune responses. TLR specificity and activation are strictly and finely tuned at multiple levels of various signal transduction pathways, resulting in complex signaling platforms. Many molecules, ranging from membrane and cytosol to nuclear, contribute to TLR ligand discrimination or receptor signaling and play different roles in the regulation of TLR responses via different mechanisms, such as cross-regulation, protein modification, helper cofactors, and posttranscriptional and epigenetic regulation. Herein, we summarize the most recent literature that provides new insight into regulation of TLR signaling-triggered innate immune responses. A greater understanding of the mechanisms underlying the control of TLR signaling may provide new targets for therapeutic intervention for infections and inflammatory diseases.

Keywords: TLR signaling; immune regulation; innate immunity; inflammation

Introduction

Innate immunity—considered to be a sentinel for the immune system—is initiated through the activation of pattern recognition receptors (PRRs) by pathogenic or endogenous motifs. Innate immune cells express various PRRs, and Toll-like receptors (TLRs) are the best characterized PRRs.[1] TLRs trigger innate immune responses by activating signaling pathways dependent on the adaptors MyD88 or TRIF, and then sequentially induce the release of proinflammatory cytokines, type I interferon, chemokines, and antimicrobial proteins. This initial immune defense against foreign and dangerous material is also critical for mounting appropriate acquired immune responses. TLR signaling is well regulated, positively and negatively, to prevent inappropriate activation or overactivation that might cause damaging inflammation to the host. A number of endogenous molecules present in normal individuals also exert regulatory effects that help to avoid excessive or uncontrolled inflammation-inducing signaling. To date, the regulation of TLR function has been the subject of intensive research, with various signaling molecules having been shown to exert regulation of TLR pathways to maintain immunological balance. In the present review, we will focus on recent advances in the study of TLR biology, and highlight the modulation at multiple levels of signaling by TLR-triggered innate immune responses (Fig. 1).

Structure and localization of TLRs

Type I transmembrane proteins, the TLR family has been described as a major class of PRRs with a critical role in the innate immune system. To date, 10 functional TLRs (TLR1 to TLR10) have been identified in humans, while 12 TLRs (TLR1 to TLR9 and TLR11 to TLR13) have been

doi: 10.1111/j.1749-6632.2012.06786.x

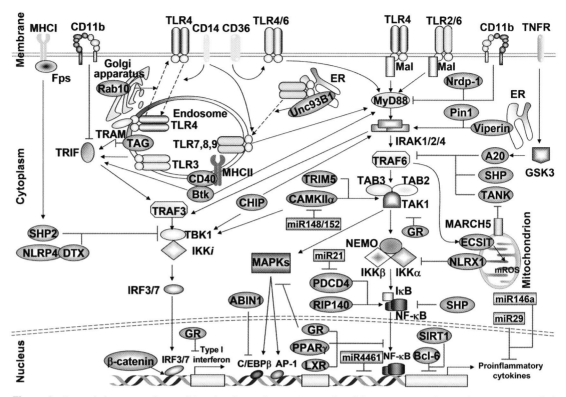

Figure 1. Currently known regulators of TLR signaling pathways. TLR-mediated downstream signaling pathways are controlled mainly by MyD88, which is used by all TLRs except TLR3, and TRIF, which is used by TLR3 and TLR4. TLR signaling can be controlled by membrane-associated regulators, such as CD14, CD11b, MHC II, TNFR, and CD36. The next line of defense against TLR-mediated overresponses is through several intracellular regulators. Ubiquin-modifying enzymes Nrdp-1, CHIP (in complex with PKCζ and Src), A20, TRIM5, and DTX (recruited by NLRP4) are reported to be responsible for negative or positive regulation of molecules associated with TLR signaling. MHC II and TAG in endosomes, TANK (catalyzed by MARCH5) and ECSIT, as well as NLRX1, in mitochondria, Unc93B1 and viperin on ER, and Rab10 in the Golgi apparatus also participate in TLR-triggered innate immune responses. Helper cofactors such as GR, LXR, PPARγ, SHP, RIP140, Pin1, TANK, and ABIN1 have been identified as pivotal regulators. MiRNA-21, miRNA-148/152, miRNA-466l, miRNA-29, and miRNA-146a have been described to control gene expression of TLR signaling at the posttranscriptional level. β-catenin, SIRT1, and Bcl-6 epigenetically fine-tune distinct functional sets of TLR-associated genes.

identified in mice.[2] TLRs are responsible for sensing invading pathogens in different parts of a cell, such as the plasma membrane (TLR1, TLR2, TLR4, TLR5, TLR6, and TLR11) or in intracellular endosomes and lysosomes (TLR3, TLR7, TLR8, TLR9, and TLR10). Except for TLR5, which recognizes flagellin, cell-surface TLRs recognize microbial membrane lipids, while TLRs that reside in intracellular organelles recognize microbial nucleic acids. In addition to microbial ligands, TLRs have been found to respond to endogenous host molecules and to trigger inflammatory responses. Most endogenous TLR ligands are produced as danger signals during inflammation and tissue injury, or by tumor cells. They include degradation products of high-mobility group box 1 (HMGB1) proteins, heat–shock proteins, extracellular matrix (ECM), chromatin-DNA, ribonucleoprotein complexes, and immune complex.[3]

TLR signaling pathway

TLRs are characterized with a cytoplasmic Toll/IL-1R homology (TIR) domain.[4] Upon ligand stimulation TLRs recruit different adaptor proteins, such as MyD88, Mal, TRAM, and TRIF, through specific TIR–TIR interactions. Except for TLR3, most TLRs recruit MyD88 and initiate a MyD88-dependent signaling pathway upon stimulation with TLR agonists. TLR2 and TLR4 signaling, in addition, requires the cooperation of the adaptor Mal, which facilitates the interaction between MyD88 and activated TLRs to initiate signal transduction. Engagement of MyD88 activates IL-1RI–associated protein kinases (IRAKs), resulting in an interaction with tumor necrosis factor receptor–associated factor 6 (TRAF6). TRAF6, an E3 ubiquitin ligase, catalyzes formation of a complex of Ubc13 and Uev1A, which in turn activates the TAK1/TAB1/TAB2/3 complex that subsequently phosphorylates IκB kinase (IKK)-β and MAP kinase (MAPKs). Activation of a complex composed of IKK-α, IKK-β, and NEMO (NF-κB essential modulator) results in the degradation of IκB, allowing NF-κB translocation to the nucleus and induction of transcription of NF-κB target genes. Simultaneously, MAP kinase activation is critical for activation of AP-1, and thus production of inflammatory cytokines.

TLR3 and TLR4 activate TRIF-dependent (MyD88-independent pathway) signaling. The interaction between TLR4 and TRIF requires the adaptor TRAM, and TRIF recruits TRAF6 or RIP1 to activate NF-κB, similar to the MyD88-dependent pathway. TRIF recruits another signaling complex composed of TRAF3/TBK1/IKK-i to phosphorylate interferon-regulatory factor 3 (IRF3), which induces expression of type I IFN genes.[5]

Membrane-associated regulators of TLR signaling

As mentioned above, TLR2 forms heterodimers with TLR1 or TLR6, which leads to the speculation that combinatorial signaling among other TLRs might account for the breadth of activity of this family of receptors. The recent identification of coreceptors that modulate TLR function suggests an emerging paradigm in which TLRs act together with other cell surface molecules to bridge microbial or modified endogenous ligand recognition and crosstalk of TLR-dependent signaling pathways.[2]

As one example of a coreceptor, CD14 is a glycosylphosphatidylinositol-anchored protein that forms a horseshoe-shaped structure that is similar to the TLR ectodomains. CD14 chaperones lipopolysaccharide (LPS) from the LPS-binding protein (LBP) to the TLR4–MD2 complex at the cell surface; it also mediates TNF-α and IL-6 production in response to TLR4 and TLR2–TLR6 ligands. Recent work has shown that CD14 induces a Syk/PLCγ2-dependent endocytosis pathway that promotes the internalization of TLR4 and TRIF-dependent signaling that induces IFN-γ expression.[6] CD14 also constitutively interacts with MyD88-dependent TLR7 and TLR9 and is necessary for induction of proinflammatory cytokines.[7]

Another example is the main β_2 integrin receptor for fibrinogen Mac-1 (CD11b-CD18; $\alpha_M\beta_2$; CR3), which is highly expressed on innate cells and participates in cell activation, chemotaxis, cytotoxicity, and phagocytosis. High-avidity ligation of ITAM-coupled β_2 integrins and FcγRs has been reported to indirectly inhibit LPS-induced expression of IL-6 and TNF-α mRNA through production of IL-10, together with the inhibitory molecules A20, SOCS3, ABIN, STAT3, and Hes1.[8] Recently, we identified an unexpected role for integrin CD11b in negative regulation of TLR-triggered inflammatory responses by activating Syk and promoting degradation of MyD88 and TRIF via Cbl-b. This is evidence for CD11b as a negative regulator of the TLR signal pathway by engaging in direct crosstalk with the TLR signaling pathway.[9]

Major histocompatibility complex (MHC) class I molecules are heterodimers composed of a membrane-bound heavy chain and β_2-microglobulin (β_2m). MHC class I molecules can form complexes on the cell surface with small-peptide fragments of endogenously produced antigens and present them to CD8+ cytotoxic T lymphocytes. Recently, we demonstrated a previously unknown, nonclassical function of constitutively expressed membrane MHC class I molecules, which is to crosstalk with TLR signaling via reverse signaling. The intracellular domain of MHC class I molecules can be phosphorylated by Src kinase as a result of TLR activation; phosophorylated MHC class I then interacts directly with the tyrosine kinase Fps. Fps then recruits the phosphatase SHP-2, which, mediated by TRAF6 and TANK-binding kinase1 (TBK1), interferes with TLR signaling and, finally, suppresses innate inflammatory responses.[10]

TNF receptors (TNFRs) induce feedback inhibition that would be particularly important to restrain and fine-tune inflammation. A study by Park et al. has shown that TNF-α–induced cross-tolerization is mediated by attenuated TLR4-induced signaling and suppressed chromatin remodeling by GSK3, which augments negative feedback by the signaling inhibitors A20 and IκBα.[11]

CD36 is found in lipid rafts as the class B scavenger receptor that binds polyanionic ligands of both pathogen and self origin. Recently, CD36 was identified to act as a new coreceptor for oxidized low-density lipoprotein (LDL) and amyloid-β peptide, and to facilitate assembly of previously undescribed TLR4/6 heterodimer through Src kinases, leading to the regulation of TLR signaling.[12]

Intracellular regulators of TLR signaling

Various intracellular signaling molecules have been shown to be involved in the tight regulation of the TLR pathway to maintain the immunological balance.

Ubiquin-modifying enzymes
The processes of protein ubiquitination mediated by E3 ubiquitin ligase and of protein deubiquitination mediated by deubiquitylating enzymes (DUBs) have been shown to provide specificity and to regulate the intensity of TLR signaling pathways. Recently, Nrdp-1, a novel E3 ligase, has been shown to be an important modulator of TLR signaling pathways. Nrdp-1 directly binds and polyubiquitinates MyD88 and TBK1, which induces MyD88 degradation, to attenuate production of inflammatory cytokines, and enhances TBK1 activation, to promote preferential type I IFN production.[13]

Our recent study provides new insight into the unexpected role of the carboxyl terminus of constitutive heat shock cognate 70 (HSC70)-interacting protein (CHIP, also known as Stub1) in promoting TLR-triggered innate immune responses.[14] CHIP can facilitate the formation of a TLR signaling complex by recruiting, polyubiquitinating, and activating tyrosine kinase Src and atypical protein kinase Cζ (PKCζ), thereby leading to activation of IRAK1, TBK1, and IRF3/7.[14]

A recent study by Shembade et al. has indicated that the zinc finger protein A20, which contains deubiquitinase and E3 ligase domains, functions as a ubiquitin-editing enzyme downstream of TLRs. A20 inhibits the E3 ligase activities of TRAF6, TRAF2, and cIAP1 by antagonizing interactions with the E2 ubiquitin conjugating enzymes Ubc13 and UbcH5c, and thus negatively regulates inflammation.[15]

Pertel et al. have reported that TRIM5, a RING domain-E3 ubiquitin ligase, catalyzes the synthesis of unattached K63-linked ubiquitin chains that activate the TAK1 kinase complex and stimulate AP-1 and NF-κB signaling, thus playing a general role in cellular responses to LPS.[16]

More recently, a study by Cui et al. identified NLRP4 as a molecule required for the regulation of TLR3-triggered type I interferon signaling by recruiting the E3 ubiquitin ligase DTX4 to TBK1 for Lys-48 (K48)-linked polyubiquitination at Lys-670, leading to degradation of TBK1.[17]

Subcellular organelle regulators of TLR signaling

Within a cell the major subcellular organelles include endosomes, mitochondria, the endoplasmic reticulum (ER), and the Golgi apparatus, each with specialized structures and specific functions. Recognition of pathogen-associated molecular patterns (PAMPs) by TLRs (TLR3/7/8/9 and probably TLR4) inside the endosome as well as ER controls the transport of TLRs to their appropriate locations. In addition to their well-appreciated roles in cellular metabolism and programmed cell death, mitochondria also participate in TLR-triggered innate immune responses.

Regulators in endosomes
Upon activation, TLR3 and TLR9, on the ER membrane, and TLR4, on the cell surface, translocate into endosomes. In endosomes, TLRs initiate downstream signal transduction in either a MyD88- or TRIF-dependent manner. A recent report provides new insight into nonclassical functions of the intracellular MHC class II molecules, which are also abundant in the endosomal compartment, by promoting full activation of TLR-triggered innate immune responses. Intracellular MHC class II molecules can function as adaptors that interact with the tyrosine kinase Btk via the costimulatory molecule CD40, which maintains Btk activation after stimulation with TLR ligands. Activated Btk interacts with the adaptor molecules MyD88 and TRIF that leads to enhanced production of proinflammatory cytokines and type I interferons.[18] A splice variant of TRAM, TAG (TRAM adaptor with GOLD domain), has also been shown to localize in late endosomes positive for the GTPase Rab7a after stimulation with LPS, and displace the adaptor TRIF from TRAM to inhibit the MyD88-independent pathway.[19]

Regulators in the mitochondrion

The mitochondrion is rapidly emerging as an important platform for TLR signaling. It has been recently revealed that the mitochondrial protein MARCH5 is a novel positive regulator of TLR7 signaling. MARCH5 catalyzes the K63-linked poly-ubiquitination of TANK and releases the inhibitory effects of TANK on TRAF6, thus shedding new light on the role of mitochondria in the proinflammatory response.[20] A more recent study has demonstrated that TLR signaling augments macrophage bactericidal activity through mitochondrial ROS. The activation of TLR1/2/4 initiates the recruitment of mitochondria to phagosomes allowing TRAF6 to ubiquitinate the mitochondrial protein ECSIT (evolutionarily conserved signaling intermediate in Toll pathways), which results in increased mitochondrial and cellular TLR-induced ROS generation.[21]

NOD-like receptors (NLRs) have been shown to be positive regulators of innate immune responses; however, new evidence suggests that NLRX1, predominantly expressed in mitochondria, can also act as an inhibitor of TLR-mediated responses. Xia et al. have demonstrated that NLRX1 is rapidly ubiquitinated in response to LPS stimulation, disassociates from TRAF6, and then binds directly to the IKK complex, resulting in inhibition of IKK phosphorylation and NF-κB–responsive cytokines.[22]

Regulators in the ER and Golgi apparatus

The ER luminal chaperones glucose-regulated protein of 94 kDa (GRP94) and protein associated with TLR4 A (PRAT4A) were identified to be required to mediate the proper folding of TLR1, TLR2, TLR4, TLR7, and TLR9, contributing to the idea that these TLRs can exit the ER. Recently, the novel ER-resident protein uncoordinated 93 homolog B1 (Unc93B1) was discovered to be required for the translocation of TLR7 and TLR9 to endolysosomes and to regulate excessive TLR7 activation of immune cells by employing TLR9 to counteract TLR7.[23] Antiviral protein Viperin localizes on the ER and the Golgi apparatus and is transported to the cytoplasmic lipid-enriched compartments called lipid droplets. A recent study has shown that Viperin, induced after TLR7 or TLR9 stimulation, interacts with IRAK1 and TRAF6 to recruit them to lipid bodies and to facilitate K63-linked ubiquitination of IRAK1, leading to IRF7 activation and type I IFN production by pDCs.[24] TLR4 cycles between the Golgi apparatus and the plasma membrane until it is engaged by LPS; this indicates that translocation of TLR4 is a regulated process that may play a role in its temporal and spatial regulation. Wang et al. have recently demonstrated that the small GTPase Ras related in brain (Rab) 10 colocalizes with TLR4 in the Golgi, and facilitates TLR4 signaling by promoting replenishment of TLR4 onto the plasma membrane.[25]

Helper cofactors

Nuclear receptors are a family of ligand-dependent transcription factors that are pivotal regulators of health and disease. Endogenous and pharmacologic glucocorticoids (GCs) function via the glucocorticoid receptor (GR, a member of the nuclear hormone receptor superfamily) and have been suggested to limit the production of inflammatory mediators initiated by TLR activation via various mechanisms, including interaction with multiple signaling components such as TAK1, MAPKs, NF-κB, and AP-1.[26] A recent report demonstrated that GCs target suppressor of cytokine signaling 1 (SOCS1) and type 1 interferons to regulate TLR-induced STAT1 activation.[27] Emerging evidence suggests that nuclear receptors liver X receptors (LXRs) and peroxisome proliferator-activated receptors (PPARs) are potent inhibitors of inflammation.[28] Huang et al. have recently found that SUMOylated LXRs block TLR-induced nuclear receptor corepressor (NCoR) turnover by binding to a conserved SUMO2/SUMO3-interaction motif in coronin 2A.[29] Recent studies of combinatorial interaction of GR, LXR, and PPARγ have revealed that these nuclear receptors provide integration of responses to repress overlapping but distinct subsets of TLR target genes using nuclear receptor– and TLR-specific transrepression mechanisms.[30] The orphan nuclear receptor small heterodimer partner (SHP) was recently identified as an intrinsic negative regulator of TLR-triggered inflammatory responses. SHP expression is induced through activation of an AMP-activated protein kinase (AMPK) signaling pathway and then acts as both a repressor of transactivation of the NF-κB subunit p65 and an inhibitor of polyubiquitination of the adaptor TRAF6 to inhibit TLR signaling.[31]

The receptor-interacting protein RIP140 can act as corepressor or coactivator of various transcription factors and nuclear receptors and has dual regulatory functions in proinflammatory cytokine production. RIP140 degradation has also been described to play an important role in resolving inflammation and endotoxin tolerance. LPS activates Syk-mediated phosphorylation and ubiquitination of RIP140 and promotes the interaction of the NF-κB subunit RelA with RIP140, leading to recruitment of the E3 ligase SCF, which degrades RIP140 to inactivate genes encoding inflammatory cytokines.[32]

The prolyl isomerase Pin1 is the only known phosphorylation-specific isomerase that controls the function of many key regulators in various cellular processes. A study by Tun-Kyi *et al.* has described the essential role for Pin1 in TLR signaling and type I interferon–mediated immunity. Activated by TLR7 and TLR9 agonists, Pin1 binds and activates IRAK1 and subsequently facilitates its release from the receptor complex to activate the transcription factor IRF7 and to induce type I interferon.[33]

TRAF family member–associated NF-κB activator (TANK) has been implicated in positive regulation of IRF3 as well as NF-κB, while it was recently identified as a negative regulator of proinflammatory cytokine production induced by TLR signaling by controlling TRAF ubiquitination *in vivo*.[34]

A20-binding inhibitor of NF-κB (ABIN1) has recently been shown to act as an essential anti-inflammatory component of TLR signaling, which controls TLR-mediated CCAAT/enhancer-binding protein β (C/EBPβ) activation and protects from inflammatory disease.[35]

Epigenetic regulation of TLR signaling

Major epigenetic events and activities include small noncoding RNAs, DNA methylation, histone modification, and chromation remodeling, all of which provide additional layers of transcription regulation and have been discovered to play fundamental roles in gene expression following environmental stimuli.

Posttranscriptional regulation of miRNAs
Regulation of TLR signaling pathway by the recently identified class of noncoding small RNA molecules known as miRNAs is an emerging area of research. New miRNAs have been described to control gene expression at the posttranscriptional level by inhibiting translation or inducing mRNA degrada-

tion.[36] Sheedy *et al.* recently identified miR-21 as a negative regulator of TLR4 signaling through the targeting of the tumor suppressor PDCD4. They showed that LPS signaling via TLR4 decreased PDCD4 protein via miR-21 in a MyD88- and NF-κB–dependent manner, suggesting that this modulation regulates NF-κB activity while promoting IL-10 production.[37]

Our recent study has reported that miRNA-148/152 expression is upregulated by TLR3/4/9 agonists and subsequently targets calcium/calmodulin-dependent protein kinase II (CaMKIIα) to impair innate responses and antigen presentation of TLR-triggered dendritic cells.[38] In another study we showed that miRNA-466l upregulates IL-10 expression in TLR-triggered macrophages by antagonizing RNA-binding protein tristetraprolin (TTP)-mediated IL-10 mRNA degradation.[39] In addition, we have also reported that miRNA-29 suppresses innate immune responses to intracellular bacterial infection by directly targeting IFN-γ.[40] More recently, we have reported that CD11b selectively promotes TLR9-triggered miRNA-146a upregulation in DCs by sustaining late-phase NF-κB activation, which in turn inhibits Notch1 expression and IL-12p70 production.[41] On the other hand, TLR4-induced miR-146a supports assembly of the translation repressor complex of TNF-α by preventing the interaction of the RNA-binding protein effector Ago2 and RBM4, thus regulating both transcription silencing and translation disruption of TNF-α during TLR4-induced gene reprogramming.[42]

Epigenetic reprogramming of TLR signaling
When TLRs recognize pathogens and respond to systemic life-threatening infections, epigenetic alterations reprogram distinct functional sets of genes to both activate and repress transcription of hundreds of genes. Our recent study has described that β-catenin, activated by TLR4 and TLR3 agonists, increases IFN-β expression by binding to the C-terminal domain of the transcription factor IRF3 and recruiting the acetyltransferase p300 to the IFN-β enhanceosome via IRF3.[43] During endotoxin tolerance, initial LPS dose induces negative regulators that mediate transcription silencing upon subsequent LPS challenge. Liu *et al.* have recently reported that the energy sensor sirtuin 1 (SIRT1) is part of the master switch that coordinates

epigenetic reprogramming and shifts functional phenotypes during acute TLR4 responses and sepsis inflammation. TLR induces rapid promoter binding of NAD^+-dependent SIRT1 and then deactivates RelA/p65 through lysine 310 deacetylation, thus limiting transcription of acute proinflammatory genes.[44] Using comparative ChIP-seq analyses, Barish *et al.* found that the Bcl-6 and NF-κB cistromes mediate opposing epigenetic modifications of local chromatin in LPS-stimulated macrophages, revealing a dynamic balance between macrophage quiescence and activation via epigenetically marked *cis*-regulatory elements.[45]

Concluding remarks

The regulation of TLR-triggered innate immune responses has been intensively investigated during the past few years. TLR signaling is a tightly regulated process that is controlled at multiple levels, including posttranscriptional regulation such as ubiquitination, phosphorylation, and mRNA stability, as well as the spatial and temporal regulation of the TLRs and their signaling complexes. The present focus of the recent investigations for the new regulatory mechanisms in various aspects of TLR function have added more layers of complexity to the area of TLR signaling. Their ability to manipulate TLR activation provides both opportunities and challenges for understanding the regulation of signal transduction elicited by each TLR to achieve different physical effects. Future studies are likely to reveal more positive and negative regulators of TLR signaling, which may provide attractive therapeutic targets in infection, inflammation, autoimmune diseases, and even cancer.

Acknowledgments

We would like to thank Dr. Nan Li and Dr. Mingyue Wen for helpful discussions. This study was supported by Grants from the National Natural Science Foundation of China (30972704, 81123006), the Shanghai Rising-Star Program (A type) (12QA1404100), and from the Foundation for the Author of National Excellent Doctoral Dissertation of China (201180).

Conflicts of interest

The authors declare no conflicts of interest.

References

1. Hajishengallis, G. & J.D. Lambris. 2011. Microbial manipulation of receptor crosstalk in innate immunity. *Nat. Rev. Immunol.* **11:** 187–200.
2. Lee, C.C., A.M. Avalos & H.L. Ploegh. 2012. Accessory molecules for Toll-like receptors and their function. *Nat. Rev. Immunol.* **12:** 168–179.
3. Harris, H.E., U. Andersson & D.S. Pisetsky. 2012. HMGB1: a multifunctional alarmin driving autoimmune and inflammatory disease. *Nat. Rev. Rheumatol.* **8:** 195–202.
4. Takeuchi, O. & S. Akira. 2010. Pattern recognition receptors and inflammation. *Cell* **140:** 805–820.
5. Kawai, T. & S. Akira. 2010. The role of pattern-recognition receptors in innate immunity: update on Toll-like receptors. *Nat. Immunol.* **11:** 373–384.
6. Zanoni, I. *et al.* 2011. CD14 controls the LPS-induced endocytosis of Toll-like receptor 4. *Cell* **147:** 868–880.
7. Baumann, C.L. *et al.* 2010. CD14 is a coreceptor of Toll-like receptors 7 and 9. *J. Exp. Med.* **207:** 2689–2701.
8. Wang, L. *et al.* 2010. Indirect inhibition of Toll-like receptor and type I interferon responses by ITAM-coupled receptors and integrins. *Immunity* **32:** 518–530.
9. Han, C. *et al.* 2010. Integrin CD11b negatively regulates TLR-triggered inflammatory responses by activating Syk and promoting degradation of MyD88 and TRIF via Cbl-b. *Nat. Immunol.* **11:** 734–742.
10. Xu, S. *et al.* 2012. Constitutive MHC class I molecules negatively regulate TLR-triggered inflammatory responses via the Fps-SHP-2 pathway. *Nat. Immunol.* **13:** 551–559.
11. Park, S.H., K.H. Park-Min, J. Chen, *et al.* 2011. Tumor necrosis factor induces GSK3 kinase-mediated cross-tolerance to endotoxin in macrophages. *Nat. Immunol.* **12:** 607–615.
12. Stewart, C.R. *et al.* 2010. CD36 ligands promote sterile inflammation through assembly of a Toll-like receptor 4 and 6 heterodimer. *Nat. Immunol.* **11:** 155–161.
13. Wang, C. *et al.* 2009. The E3 ubiquitin ligase Nrdp1 'preferentially' promotes TLR-mediated production of type I interferon. *Nat. Immunol.* **10:** 744–752.
14. Yang, M. *et al.* 2011. E3 ubiquitin ligase CHIP facilitates Toll-like receptor signaling by recruiting and polyubiquitinating Src and atypical PKCζ. *J. Exp. Med.* **208:** 2099–2112.
15. Shembade, N., A. Ma & E.W. Harhaj. 2010. Inhibition of NF-kappaB signaling by A20 through disruption of ubiquitin enzyme complexes. *Science* **327:** 1135–1139.
16. Pertel, T. *et al.* 2011. TRIM5 is an innate immune sensor for the retrovirus capsid lattice. *Nature* **472:** 361–365.
17. Cui, J. *et al.* 2012. NLRP4 negatively regulates type I interferon signaling by targeting the kinase TBK1 for degradation via the ubiquitin ligase DTX4. *Nat. Immunol.* **13:** 387–395.
18. Liu, X. *et al.* 2011. Intracellular MHC class II molecules promote TLR-triggered innate immune responses by maintaining activation of the kinase Btk. *Nat. Immunol.* **12:** 416–424.
19. Palsson-McDermott, E.M. *et al.* 2009. TAG, a splice variant of the adaptor TRAM, negatively regulates the adaptor MyD88-independent TLR4 pathway. *Nat. Immunol.* **10:** 579–586.
20. Shi, H.X. *et al.* 2011. Mitochondrial ubiquitin ligase MARCH5 promotes TLR7 signaling by attenuating TANK action. *PLoS Pathog.* **7:** 1–15.

21. West, A.P. *et al.* 2011. TLR signalling augments macrophage bactericidal activity through mitochondrial ROS. *Nature* **472:** 476–480.

22. Xia, X. *et al.* 2011. NLRX1 negatively regulates TLR-induced NF-kappaB signaling by targeting TRAF6 and IKK. *Immunity* **34:** 843–853.

23. Fukui, R. *et al.* 2011. Unc93B1 restricts systemic lethal inflammation by orchestrating Toll-like receptor 7 and 9 trafficking. *Immunity* **35:** 69–81.

24. Saitoh, T. *et al.* 2011. Antiviral protein Viperin promotes Toll-like receptor 7- and Toll-like receptor 9-mediated type I interferon production in plasmacytoid dendritic cells. *Immunity* **34:** 352–363.

25. Wang, D. *et al.* 2010. Ras-related protein Rab10 facilitates TLR4 signaling by promoting replenishment of TLR4 onto the plasma membrane. *Proc. Natl. Acad. Sci. USA* **107:** 13806–13811.

26. Bhattacharyya, S. *et al.* 2010. TAK1 targeting by glucocorticoids determines JNK and IκB regulation in Toll-like receptor–stimulated macrophages. *Blood* **115:** 1921–1931.

27. Bhattacharyya, S. *et al.* 2011. Glucocorticoids target suppressor of cytokine signaling 1 (SOCS1) and type 1 interferons to regulate Toll-like receptor–induced STAT1 activation. *Proc. Natl. Acad. Sci. USA* **108:** 9554–9559.

28. Yoko, K. & J.B. Steven. 2012. Liver X receptor and peroxisome proliferator-activated receptor as integrators of lipid homeostasis and immunity. *Immunol. Rev.* **249:** 72–83.

29. Wendy, H. *et al.* 2011. Coronin 2A mediates actin-dependent de-repression of inflammatory response genes. *Nature* **470:** 414–418.

30. Ogawa, S. *et al.* 2005. Molecular determinants of crosstalk between nuclear receptors and toll-like receptors. *Cell* **122:** 707–721.

31. Yuk, J.M. *et al.* 2011. The orphan nuclear receptor SHP acts as a negative regulator in inflammatory signaling triggered by Toll-like receptors. *Nat. Immunol.* **12:** 742–751.

32. Ho, P.C. *et al.* 2012. NF-kappaB-mediated degradation of the coactivator RIP140 regulates inflammatory responses and contributes to endotoxin tolerance. *Nat. Immunol.* **13:** 379–386.

33. Tun-Kyi, A. *et al.* 2011. Essential role for the prolyl isomerase Pin1 in Toll-like receptor signaling and type I interferon-mediated immunity. *Nat. Immunol.* **12:** 733–741.

34. Kawagoe, T. *et al.* 2009. TANK is a negative regulator of Toll-like receptor signaling and is critical for the prevention of autoimmune nephritis. *Nat. Immunol.* **10:** 965–972.

35. Zhou, J. *et al.* 2011. A20-binding inhibitor of NF-kappaB (ABIN1) controls Toll-like receptor-mediated CCAAT/enhancer-binding protein beta activation and protects from inflammatory disease. *Proc. Natl. Acad. Sci. USA* **108:** 998–1006.

36. O'Neill, L.A., F.J. Sheedy & C.E. McCoy. 2011. MicroRNAs: the fine-tuners of Toll-like receptor signalling. *Nat. Rev. Immunol.* **11:** 163–175.

37. Sheedy, F.J. *et al.* 2010. Negative regulation of TLR4 via targeting of the proinflammatory tumor suppressor PDCD4 by the microRNA miR-21. *Nat. Immunol.* **11:** 141–147.

38. Liu, X. *et al.* 2010. MicroRNA-148/152 impair innate response and antigen presentation of TLR-triggered dendritic cells by targeting CaMKIIalpha. *J. Immunol.* **185:** 7244–7251.

39. Ma, F. *et al.* 2010. MicroRNA-466l upregulates IL-10 expression in TLR-triggered macrophages by antagonizing RNA-binding protein tristetraprolin-mediated IL-10 mRNA degradation. *J. Immunol.* **184:** 6053–6059.

40. Ma, F. *et al.* 2011. The microRNA miR-29 controls innate and adaptive immune responses to intracellular bacterial infection by targeting interferon-gamma. *Nat. Immunol.* **12:** 861–869.

41. Bai, Y. *et al.* 2012. Integrin CD11b negatively regulates TLR9-triggered dendritic cell cross-priming by upregulating microRNA-146a. *J. Immunol.* **188:** 5293–5302.

42. El, G.M. *et al.* 2011. MicroRNA-146a regulates both transcription silencing and translation disruption of TNF-alpha during TLR4-induced gene reprogramming. *J. Leukoc. Biol.* **90:** 509–519.

43. Yang, P. *et al.* 2010. The cytosolic nucleic acid sensor LRRFIP1 mediates the production of type I interferon via a beta-catenin-dependent pathway. *Nat. Immunol.* **11:** 487–494.

44. Liu, T.F. *et al.* 2011. NAD+-dependent SIRT1 deacetylase participates in epigenetic reprogramming during endotoxin tolerance. *J. Biol. Chem.* **286:** 9856–9864.

45. Barish, G.D. *et al.* 2010. Bcl-6 and NF-kappaB cistromes mediate opposing regulation of the innate immune response. *Genes Dev.* **24:** 2760–2765.

Ann. N.Y. Acad. Sci. ISSN 0077-8923

ANNALS OF THE NEW YORK ACADEMY OF SCIENCES

Issue: *Translational Immunology in Asia-Oceania*

TAP expression level in tumor cells defines the nature and processing of MHC class I peptides for recognition by tumor-specific cytotoxic T lymphocytes

Faten El Hage,[1] Aurélie Durgeau,[2] and Fathia Mami-Chouaib[2]

[1]Chimie et Sciences de la Vie et de la Terre, Université Saint-Esprit de Kaslik, Jounieh, Lebanon. [2]Integrated Research Cancer Institute in Villejuif, Institut de Cancérologie Gustave Roussy, Villejuif, France

Address for correspondence: Fathia Mami-Chouaib, Inserm U753, Institut de Cancérologie Gustave Roussy (IGR), 114 rue Édouard Vaillant, IGR, F-94805 Villejuif, France. cfathia@igr.fr

We identified that the antigen preprocalcitonin (ppCT) is recognized on a human lung carcinoma by a cytotoxic T lymphocyte clone derived from autologous tumor-infiltrating lymphocytes. The antigenic peptide ppCT$_{16-25}$ is encoded by the gene calcitonin-related polypeptide alpha (*CALCA*), which codes for CT and is overexpressed in several lung carcinomas compared with normal tissues. The ppCT peptide is derived from the C-terminal region of the signal peptide and is processed independently of proteasomes and the transporter associated with antigen processing (TAP)1/TAP2 heterodimeric complexes. Instead, processing occurs within the endoplasmic reticulum by a novel mechanism involving signal pepsidase (SP) and signal peptide peptidase (SPP). Although lung cancer cells bearing the ppCT$_{16-25}$ epitope displayed low levels of TAP, restoration of TAP expression by interferon (IFN)-γ treatment or by *TAP1/TAP2* gene transfer inhibited ppCT antigen presentation. Thus, the ppCT$_{16-25}$ human tumor epitope requires low TAP expression for efficient presentation. These results indicate that emerging SP-generated peptides represent alternative T cell targets that permit cytotoxic T lymphocytes to destroy TAP-impaired tumors, a process that helps to overcome tumor escape from CD8$^+$ T cell immunity. Additionally, our data suggest that ppCT is a promising candidate for cancer immunotherapy.

Keywords: lung cancer; tumor-associated antigens; cytotoxic T lymphocytes; antigen processing

Introduction

Cytotoxic T lymphocytes (CTLs) correspond to major effectors in host defense against malignant transformation. Killing of cancer cells by CD8$^+$ T cells is triggered following interaction of T cell receptor (TCR) with the specific tumor peptide–major histocompatibility complex class I molecule (MHC-I) complex. A large number of tumor-associated antigens (TAAs) recognized by CTLs have been identified, primarily in melanoma. With regard to lung cancer, the identified T cell target antigens include peptides encoded by the HER2/neu proto-oncogene[1] and the *MUC1* gene[2]—which are overexpressed in many lung tumors—and by several genes that were found to contain a point mutation in tumor cells compared to autologous normal cells. These mutated genes include elongation factor 2,[3] malic enzyme,[4] α-actinin-4,[5] and nuclear tran-

scription factor Y subunit gamma (NFYC).[6] Moreover, several cancer/germline genes are expressed in lung cancer, which should lead to the presence of tumor-specific antigen at the surface of cancer cells. However, spontaneous T cell responses against the human melanoma antigen gene (MAGE)-type antigens have thus far not been observed in lung cancer patients. Therefore, identification of new human lung cancer antigens, in particular those shared by several tumors, would help in the design of novel vaccination approaches in lung cancer.

Preprocalcitonin is a shared lung tumor-associated antigen

Lung cancer includes small cell lung carcinomas (SCLC), non-small cell lung carcinomas (NSCLC), and a large group that comprises squamous-cell (SCC), adeno- (ADC), and large-cell (LCC) carcinomas. From a LCC we previously established

doi: 10.1111/j.1749-6632.2012.06777.x

a tumor cell line (IGR-Heu), and from tumor-infiltrating lymphocytes (TILs) we isolated a CTL clone (Heu161) able to lyse autologous cancer cells in an HLA-A2–restricted manner. Using a genetic method based on the generation of a cDNA library from tumor cells and screening with specific T lymphocytes, we identified the antigens recognized by the T cell clone. The antigen preprocalcitonin (ppCT) is encoded by the gene calcitonin-related polypeptide alpha (*CALCA*), which codes for calcitonin (CT) and for α-calcitonin gene–related peptide (α-CGRP). *CALCA* includes five introns and six exons;[7] exons 1, 2, 3, and 4 are joined to produce the *CT* mRNA in thyroid C cells, while exons 1, 2, 3, 5, and 6 form the α-*CGRP* mRNA in neuronal cells. CT is a hormone involved in protecting the skeleton during periods of calcium stress. In humans, CT is synthesized as a precursor protein, ppCT, which includes a signal sequence of 25 aa and proCT, the latter consisting of an N-terminal region, CT itself (32 aa), and a C-terminal peptide.[7]

CT is known to be produced at high levels by medullary thyroid carcinoma (MTC) and, more surprisingly, by some lung carcinomas.[8] Using quantitative RT-PCR, we demonstrated that *CALCA* is overexpressed in several SCLC and NSCLC. *CALCA* overexpression has also been reported in prostate cancer.[9] In addition, hypercalcemia resulting from an increase in CT plasma levels was observed in several patients with different types of cancers, including breast cancer, pancreatic cancer, liver cancer, and leukemia. The mechanisms leading to overexpression of CT in these cancers are not yet well understood. Silencing of tumor suppressors or other cancer-associated genes by methylation of CpG islands located in the gene promoter and/or 5′ region is a common feature of human tumors. In MTC, one 5′ region of *CALCA* was found to be hypomethylated.[10] Moreover, the methylation of this 5′ region correlated with decreased expression in most tissues. However, in lung cancer, methylation of the *CALCA* promoter and 5′ region did not correlate with inhibition of expression, but rather with induction of its transcription.[10]

CTL epitope from ppCT signal sequence is processed by SP and SPP

Most antigenic peptides recognized by CD8[+] T cells are derived from degradation of intracellular mature proteins by proteasomes and translocation to the lumen of the endoplasmic reticulum (ER) by the transporter associated with antigen processing (TAP)1/TAP2 heterodimeric complex. The resulting 8–10 aa peptides are then loaded onto MHC-I molecules and conveyed to the surface of antigen-presenting cells (APC) or target cells for T cell recognition. Defects in processing molecules, such as in the proteasome or TAP subunits, have been described as a strategy used by tumor cells to counter the host T cell response. Indeed, TAP deficiencies have also been observed in a wide variety of human cancers, including cervical carcinoma, head and neck carcinoma, melanoma, and gastric cancer, and are associated with tumor escape from the immune system.

An increasing number of epitopes recognized by tumor-reactive T cells have been reported to result from nonclassical mechanisms acting at the transcription, splicing, or translational levels. Indeed, proteasome-TAP–independent tumor-specific CD8[+] T cell epitopes generated either by the cytosolic metallopeptidase insulin-degrading enzyme or the cytosolic endopeptidases nardilysin and thimet oligopeptidase have been identified.[11] Proteasome-TAP–independent presentation of peptides can also be mediated by the secretory pathway in which the proteolytic enzyme furin releases C-terminal peptides.[12] Moreover, CTL specific for antigen-processing mutants have been described in humans and mouse models, and were found to recognize epitopes processed by a TAP-independent mechanism. Peptide elution experiments indicated that these epitopes can be derived from signal sequences of cellular proteins.[13] Among signal peptide-derived tumor epitopes, melanoma-associated tyrosinase peptides 1–9 is presented independently of TAP and proteasomes.[14] However, little is known of the exact processing mechanisms of these antigenic peptides. We have demonstrated that the signal sequence of the CT and α-CGRP preprohormones contains an antigenic peptide that can be specifically recognized by CTL, such as the Heu161 clone, on the lung tumor or MTC cells expressing *CALCA*.

Like other proteins, the leader sequence of ppCT is markedly hydrophobic and mediates binding of the protein precursor to the membrane of the ER; the leader sequence is then immediately cleaved at its C-terminal region by SP.[15] After release from precursor proteins, signal peptides with a

A

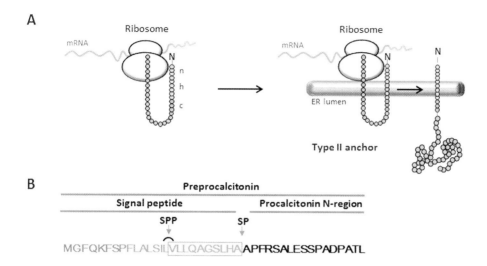

B

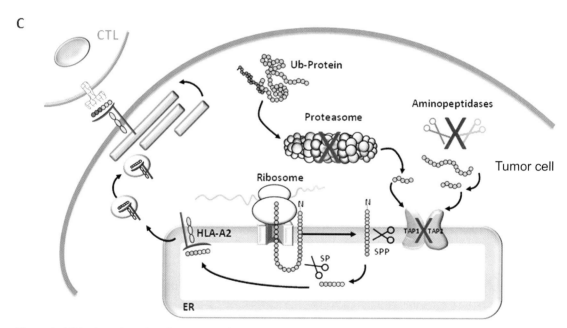

Figure 1. (A) Anchor orientation of a type II signal peptide. A signal peptide is formed by two hydrophilic cores (c and n) separated by a hydrophobic region (h). A type II anchor has its N-terminal region in the cytoplasm.[16] (B) Structure of the ppCT N-terminal region. The ppCT$_{16-25}$ epitope (boxed) is located at the C-terminus of the CT hormone precursor signal sequence. Arrows indicate the SP and the approximate SPP cleavage sites. (C) Processing of the ppCT$_{16-25}$ antigenic peptide. The processing of ppCT$_{16-25}$ epitope is independent of cytoplasmic aminopeptidases and proteasome-TAP pathway. It occurs within the ER by SP and SPP. The resulting peptide is then loaded on HLA-A2 molecules and conveyed to the surface of tumor cells for T cell recognition.

type II orientation, that is, those spanning the ER membrane with the n region exposed toward the cytosol and the c region facing the ER lumen[16] (Fig. 1A), can undergo intramembrane proteolysis and be cleaved in the center of their h region by the aspartic protease the signal peptide peptidase (SPP).[17] After cleavage by SPP, signal peptide fragments can be released either into the cytoplasm, to be processed by the proteasome-TAP pathway,[18] or the ER, where they follow TAP-independent processing.[16] Our results indicate that the ppCT signal peptide has a type II orientation (Fig. 1A), is a substrate of SPP, and that SPP cleaves the $ppCT_{16-25}$ CTL epitope at its N-terminal region, while the SP cleaves its C-terminal region (Fig. 1B). This CTL epitope derives from the C-terminus of the ppCT signal sequence; it is therefore probably released directly into the ER and, therefore, does not require proteasomes and TAP for its processing (Fig. 1C).[19]

TAP expression level in cancer cells regulates preprocalcitonin epitope presentation

Using quantitative reverse transcription polymerase chain reaction (RT-PCR) and Western blot analyses, we showed that several human lung cancer cell lines and primary tumors display weak expression of TAP1 molecules. TAP downregulation has also been observed in several SCLC and NSCLC specimens by immunohistochemical analysis. This suggested that human lung cancers represent poor targets for MHC-I–restricted CTL and thus correspond to poor candidates for TAA-based immunotherapy. However, our data indicated that tumor antigen can be presented on cancer cells following degradation by at least two parallel mechanisms (that is, proteasome–TAP or SP–SPP), which together contribute to the diversity of antigenic peptides displayed at the surface of malignant cells. The $ppCT_{16-25}$ antigenic peptide is the first molecularly characterized human T cell epitope associated with impaired peptide processing (TEIPP). Indeed, the NSCLC cell line bearing this epitope exhibited low levels of TAP1 and TAP2, and downregulation of TAP is required for CTL recognition. Moreover, our results indicated that siRNA knockdown of TAP in ppCT-expressing allogeneic cancer cells resulted in their increased recognition by ppCT-specific T cells.[20] These data suggest that peptides derived from signal sequences of available secreted self-proteins and processed by the SP–SPP pathway represent a substantial pool of epitopes presented by TAP-deficient tumors.

Peptides derived from signal sequences contribute to stabilizing MHC molecules in TAP-deficient cells, even though the expression of peptide-MHC complexes remains weak. Treatment of the IGR-Heu NSCLC cell line with IFN-γ led to a decrease in ppCT peptide presentation. This is most likely due to an IFN-γ–mediated increase in TAP expression which triggered competition with other peptides entering the ER via TAP, leading to decreased loading of the ppCT peptide.[20] These data suggest that SP-processed peptides are competed away from MHC-I presentation by the large flow of TAP-transported peptides in IFN-γ–treated tumor cells. Accordingly, transduction of NSCLC cells with TAP1 and TAP2 resulted in inhibition of $ppCT_{16-25}$ epitope loading, as reflected by a decrease in target cell recognition by the specific Heu161 T cell clone. These results indicate that a competition between proteasome–TAP- and SP–SPP-dependent pathways occurs in APC and that TAP expression levels determine the antigen-processing mechanism used by cancer cells and thereby the antigenic peptide repertoire presented on their surface. They also provide evidence that peptides derived from human signal sequences only emerge at the surface of APC if there is impairment in the conventional antigen presentation pathway. Thus, emerging SP–SPP-generated peptides represent alternative T cell targets, which permit CTL to destroy TAP-impaired tumors and thereby overcome tumor escape from $CD8^+$ T cell immunity.

Preprocalcitonin is a promising target antigen for cancer immunotherapy

Although the recent identification of TAAs and clonal expansions of specific CTL clones within solid tumor infiltrates argue in favor of a role of the immune system in the control of tumor progression, it is now obvious that the development of efficient therapeutic vaccines will be long and will require the identification of additional tumor antigens and improved strategies to induce strong long-lasting CTL responses. The identification of tumor-specific epitopes as targets for antitumor CTL effectors has made possible their use in vaccination trials mainly in melanoma. With regard to lung cancer, only a few cancer vaccine trials have so far been conducted, with most of them using Mage-A3 (Ref. 21) or Mucin 1 (MUC-1)[22] antigens.

Preprocalcitonin antigen, which we have shown to induce a spontaneous CTL response in a NSCLC patient with long-term survival, and which can generate an alternative TAP-independent $CD8^+$ T cell epitope, is a promising candidate for cancer immunotherapy. Immunotherapy strategies combining both TAP-dependent and TAP-independent antigenic peptides may reinforce tumor-specific T cell responses and improve current cancer vaccines. Indeed, the presence of CTL able of eliminating both antigen processing-deficient and proficient tumors is of a major importance for the development of more efficacious anticancer immunotherapy approaches. The observation that these TAP-independent self-peptides are poorly presented by cells with normal processing status, and emerge at target cell surface only after alterations in conventional MHC-I antigen processing machinery, might explain their immunogenicity and capability to induce an efficient antitumor T cell response. Therefore, signal sequence-derived epitopes correspond to attractive candidates for specific cancer immunotherapy against TAP-impaired tumors.

Summary

We identified an antigen, ppCT, recognized on a human lung carcinoma by a CTL clone derived from autologous TILs. The antigenic peptide is presented by HLA-A2 and is encoded by the gene *CALCA*, which codes for CT and which is overexpressed in several lung carcinomas compared to normal tissues. This peptide, $ppCT_{16-25}$, is derived from the C-terminal region of the ppCT signal peptide, and is processed independently of proteasomes and TAP. Processing occurs within the ER of all tumor cells tested by a novel mechanism involving SP and SPP. Lung cancer cells bearing this epitope displayed low levels of TAP, but restoration of their expression by IFN-γ treatment or by *TAP1* and *TAP2* gene transfer inhibited ppCT antigen presentation. Thus, $ppCT_{16-25}$ is the first human tumor epitope whose surface expression requires downregulation of TAP. Lung tumors frequently display low levels of TAP and might thus be ignored by the immune system. Our results indicated that emerging SP-generated peptides represent alternative T cell targets, which permit CTL to destroy TAP-impaired tumors and thus overcome tumor escape from CD8[+] T cell immunity. ppCT is therefore a promising candidate for cancer immunotherapy.

Acknowledgments

We thank Drs. Pierre Coulie and Thorbald Van Hall for helpful discussion, and Isabelle Vergnon for technical expertise.

Conflicts of interest

The authors declare no conflicts of interest.

References

1. Yoshino, I. *et al.* 1994. HER2/neu-derived peptides are shared antigens among human non-small cell lung cancer and ovarian cancer. *Cancer Res.* **54:** 3387–3390.
2. Seregni, E. *et al.* 1996. Pattern of mucin gene expression in normal and neoplastic lung tissues. *Anticancer Res.* **16:** 2209–2213.
3. Hogan, K.T. *et al.* 1998. The peptide recognized by HLA-A68.2-restricted, squamous cell carcinoma of the lung-specific cytotoxic T lymphocytes is derived from a mutated elongation factor 2 gene. *Cancer Res.* **58:** 5144–5150.
4. Karanikas, V. *et al.* 2001. High frequency of cytolytic T lymphocytes directed against a tumor-specific mutated antigen detectable with HLA tetramers in the blood of a lung carcinoma patient with long survival. *Cancer Res.* **61:** 3718–3724.
5. Echchakir, H. *et al.* 2001. A point mutation in the alpha-actinin-4 gene generates an antigenic peptide recognized by autologous cytolytic T lymphocytes on a human lung carcinoma. *Cancer Res.* **61:** 4078–4083.
6. Takenoyama, M. *et al.* 2006. A point mutation in the NFYC gene generates an antigenic peptide recognized by autologous cytolytic T lymphocytes on a human squamous cell lung carcinoma. *Int. J. Cancer* **118:** 1992–1997.
7. Rosenfeld, M.G. *et al.* 1983. Production of a novel neuropeptide encoded by the calcitonin gene via tissue-specific RNA processing. *Nature* **304:** 129–135.
8. Bondy, P.K. 1981. The pattern of ectopic hormone production in lung cancer. *Yale J. Biol. Med.* **54:** 181–185.
9. di Sant'Agnese, P.A. & K.L. de Mesy Jensen. 1987. Neuroendocrine differentiation in prostatic carcinoma. *Hum. Pathol.* **18:** 849–856.
10. Baylin, S.B. *et al.* 1986. DNA methylation patterns of the calcitonin gene in human lung cancers and lymphomas. *Cancer Res.* **46:** 2917–2922.
11. Parmentier, N. *et al.* 2010. Production of an antigenic peptide by insulin-degrading enzyme. *Nat. Immunol.* **11:** 449–454.
12. Medina, F. *et al.* 2009. Furin-processed antigens targeted to the secretory route elicit functional TAP1$^{-/-}$ CD8[+] T lymphocytes in vivo. *J. Immunol.* **183:** 4639–4647.
13. Weinzierl, A.O. *et al.* 2008. Features of TAP-independent MHC class I ligands revealed by quantitative mass spectrometry. *Eur. J. Immunol.* **38:** 1503–1510.
14. Wolfel, C. *et al.* 2000. Transporter (TAP)- and proteasome-independent presentation of a melanoma-associated tyrosinase epitope. *Int. J. Cancer* **88:** 432–438.
15. Dalbey, R.E. *et al.* 1997. The chemistry and enzymology of the type I signal peptidases. *Protein Sci.* **6:** 1129–1138.
16. Martoglio, B. & B. Dobberstein. 1998. Signal sequences: more than just greasy peptides. *Trends Cell Biol.* **8:** 410–415.
17. Weihofen, A. *et al.* 2002. Identification of signal peptide peptidase, a presenilin-type aspartic protease. *Science* **296:** 2215–2218.
18. Bland, F.A. *et al.* 2003. Requirement of the proteasome for the trimming of signal peptide-derived epitopes presented by the nonclassical major histocompatibility complex class I molecule HLA-E. *J. Biol. Chem.* **278:** 33747–33752.

19. El Hage, F. *et al.* 2008. Preprocalcitonin signal peptide generates a cytotoxic T lymphocyte-defined tumor epitope processed by a proteasome-independent pathway. *Proc. Natl. Acad. Sci. USA.* **105:** 10119–10124.

20. Durgeau, A. *et al.* 2011. Different expression levels of the TAP peptide transporter lead to recognition of different antigenic peptides by tumor-specific CTL. *J. Immunol.* **187:** 5532–5539.

21. Brichard, V.G. & D. Lejeune. 2008. Cancer immunotherapy targeting tumour-specific antigens: towards a new therapy for minimal residual disease. *Expert Opin. Biol. Ther.* **8:** 951–968.

22. Quoix, E. *et al.* 2011. Therapeutic vaccination with TG4010 and first-line chemotherapy in advanced non-small-cell lung cancer: a controlled phase 2B trial. *Lancet Oncol.* **12:** 1125–1133.

Ann. N.Y. Acad. Sci. ISSN 0077-8923

ANNALS OF THE NEW YORK ACADEMY OF SCIENCES
Issue: *Translational Immunology in Asia-Oceania*

Proinflammatory cytokines contribute to development and function of regulatory T cells in type 1 diabetes

Helen E. Thomas,[1,2] Kate L. Graham,[1] Jonathan Chee,[1] Ranjeny Thomas,[3] Thomas W. Kay,[1,2] and Balasubramanian Krishnamurthy[1]

[1]Immunology and Diabetes Unit, St. Vincent's Institute, Fitzroy, Victoria, Australia. [2]Department of Medicine, The University of Melbourne, St. Vincent's Hospital, Fitzroy, Victoria, Australia. [3]Diamantina Institute for Cancer, Immunology, and Metabolic Medicine, University of Queensland, Princess Alexandra Hospital, Brisbane, Queensland, Australia

Address for correspondence: Dr. Helen Thomas, St. Vincent's Institute of Medical Research, 41 Victoria Parade, Fitzroy, VIC, 3065. hthomas@svi.edu.au

Type 1 diabetes is caused by immune-mediated loss of pancreatic beta cells. It has been proposed that inflammatory cytokines play a role in killing beta cells. Expression of interleukin (IL)-1 and tumor necrosis factor (TNF-α) has been detected in islets from patients with type 1 diabetes, and these cytokines can induce beta cell death *in vitro*. We produced nonobese diabetic (NOD) mice lacking receptors for these cytokines. Islets from mice lacking IL-1RI or TNFR1 were killed when transplanted into wild-type NOD mice, suggesting that cytokine action on beta cells is not required for killing. Mice lacking TNFR1 did not develop diabetes, and mice lacking IL-1R had delayed onset of diabetes, indicating a role for these cytokines in disease development. TNFR1-deficient mice had an increased number of CD4$^+$CD25$^+$FoxP3$^+$ regulatory T cells with enhanced suppressive capacity. IL-1 was produced at higher levels in NOD mice and resulted in dilution of suppressor function of CD4$^+$CD25$^+$FoxP3$^+$ regulatory T cells. Our data suggest that blocking inflammatory cytokines may increase the capacity of the immune system to suppress type 1 diabetes through regulatory T cells.

Keywords: type 1 diabetes; TNF-α; IL-1; regulatory T cells

Introduction

The incidence of type 1 diabetes, which is caused by the destruction of the insulin-producing pancreatic beta cells by autoimmune mechanisms, is increasing in many parts of the world. Disease occurs in genetically susceptible individuals, possibly triggered by an environmental event. Because it is difficult to study the disease in humans, much of what we know about type 1 diabetes comes from the nonobese diabetic (NOD) mouse model. Mice develop disease with many of the features of human diabetes.

Type 1 diabetes is characterized by loss of tolerance mechanisms that normally prevent responses to self. Strong evidence in NOD mice, and possibly in humans, indicates that insulin is the primary autoantigen recognized by autoreactive T cells.[1–3] In humans, autoantibodies to islet antigens develop and mark the onset of autoimmunity.[1] In addition, a mononuclear cell infiltrate of macrophages and T and B lymphocytes can be observed in the pancreatic islets in some humans with diabetes and in NOD mice in the preclinical phase.[4,5] Beta cell mass or function gradually declines until there is insufficient insulin production to meet metabolic demand, and then clinical signs of diabetes develop. T lymphocytes are required for destruction of beta cells, with both CD4$^+$ and CD8$^+$ T cell subsets necessary for efficient disease progression in NOD mice.

Proinflammatory cytokines

Proinflammatory cytokines including interleukin (IL)-1, tumor necrosis factor α (TNF-α), and interferon (IFN)-γ have been identified in the islets of NOD mice and humans during progression to diabetes.[6] *In vitro*, these cytokines exert cytotoxic effects on beta cells by mechanisms including production

doi: 10.1111/j.1749-6632.2012.06797.x

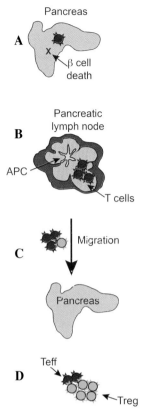

Figure 1. Mode of action of IL-1 and TNF-α in development of type 1 diabetes. We studied the effects of deficiency of IL-1 and TNF-α receptors on different steps in the pathogenesis of type 1 diabetes. (A) Beta cell death was not affected by deficiency of IL-1RI or TNFR1, nor was (B) priming and proliferation in the pancreatic lymph node. (C) Migration of autoreactive T cells to the pancreas was reduced in TNFR1-deficient NOD mice. (D) In both IL-1RI and TNFR1-deficient NOD mice there was an increase in number and/or function of CD4$^+$CD25$^+$FoxP3$^+$ T$_{reg}$ cells.

of free radicals, such as nitric oxide and reactive oxygen species, as well as activation of intracellular apoptosis pathways.[7] Because of this toxicity *in vitro*, it is widely assumed that proinflammatory cytokines cause beta cell destruction in type 1 diabetes *in vivo*. Our laboratory has systematically tested the role of these cytokines in diabetes development in NOD mice. We have made NOD mice deficient in receptors for IL-1, TNF-α, and IFN-γ and tested the effects on diabetes susceptibility.[8–10] We have found that these cytokines do not participate directly in beta cell killing *in vivo*. However, they do have a role in immune regulation and activation of immune cells. In this paper we discuss the effects of

two of these cytokines, TNF-α and IL-1, on development and function of regulatory T (T$_{reg}$) cells in the pathogenesis of type 1 diabetes.

Tumor necrosis factor

TNF-α signals through two receptors, TNFR1 and TNFR2. Most of the inflammatory effects of TNF occur through TNFR1.[11] TNFR2 is particularly highly expressed on T$_{reg}$ cells, and TNF–TNFR2 signaling promotes their expansion.[12]

Overexpression of TNF-α in the beta cells of neonatal NOD mice results in insulitis and acceleration of diabetes.[13] Likewise, blockade of TNF-α in neonatal NOD mice with anti-TNF-α antibody prevents diabetes.[14] In adult NOD mice, exogenous TNF-α delays diabetes progression, indicating the different effects of TNF-α depending on the time of administration.[15,16]

Interleukin-1

IL-1 is a proinflammatory cytokine that influences the development of many autoimmune diseases including type 1 diabetes. IL-1 signals through a heterodimeric receptor consisting of IL-1RI and the IL-1R accessory protein. IL-1β is produced in the islets of NOD mice during progression to diabetes.[6] It has been suggested that IL-1β expression results from hyperglycemia-induced inflammation resulting in NLRP3 inflammasome activation.[17] However, IL-1β expression coincides with early insulitis (four to six weeks of age), dropping off as NOD mice age and diabetes develops.[6] Therefore, it is likely that pathogen- or damage-associated molecular patterns or processes associated with islet autoreactivity but not hyperglycemia drive IL-1β overexpression during insulitis in NOD mice. In humans, IL-1 also appears to be important in early disease pathogenesis in recent onset or at-risk patients.[18,19]

TNF-α and IL-1 in diabetes development

We backcrossed mice deficient in either IL-1RI or TNFR1 to the NOD genetic background to determine the role of these cytokines in development of diabetes.[8,9] We examined the effects of cytokine receptor deficiency on T cell activation and migration to the pancreas, beta cell destruction, and development of T cell populations, in particular regulatory T cells (Fig. 1). We determined that neither IL-1 nor TNF-α are important for direct destruction of beta cells, but both are involved in development and function of regulatory T cells, with TNF-α having more of a prominent role in development of diabetes in NOD mice.

T cell activation and migration

We observed a delay in the development in diabetes in NOD mice lacking IL-1RI, but the majority of IL-1RI–deficient NOD mice developed diabetes.[9] We also did not observe any effects of IL-1RI deficiency on activation or priming of autoreactive CD8[+] T cells or on progression of insulitis. These data indicate a minor role for IL-1 in diabetes pathogenesis in NOD mice.[9]

Deficiency of TNFR1 results in complete protection from diabetes in NOD mice, a finding that we independently reproduced.[8,20] We observed a significant reduction in insulitis in the absence of TNFR1. To determine whether the CD4[+] or CD8[+] T cell compartments were involved, we crossed TNFR1-deficient NOD mice with transgenic mice expressing T cell receptor (TCR) $\alpha\beta$ chains of highly diabetogenic beta cell–specific CD4[+] (NOD4.1) and CD8[+] (NOD8.3) T cells. We observed a reduction in diabetes incidence and insulitis in both of these transgenic lines. These results indicate that both T cell compartments are affected by loss of TNFR1.[8]

While we observed a defect in homing of cells to the islets, as indicated by reduced insulitis, we did not observe an effect on priming of autoreactive T cells in the draining pancreatic lymph node in the absence of TNFR1, nor did we observe a change in expression of adhesion molecules in the pancreas of TNFR1-deficient NOD mice.[8]

Beta cell destruction

In vitro, islets are highly susceptible to killing by combinations of IL-1 + IFN-γ or TNF-α + IFN-γ.[7] This toxicity is due to upregulation of inducible nitric oxide synthase, production of free radicals, and activation of intracellular apoptosis signaling pathways.[7] Islets deficient in either IL-1RI or TNFR1 were protected from the toxic effects of cytokines *in vitro*, as expected.[8,9] To test whether TNF-α, IL-1, or both are directly involved in beta cell destruction *in vivo*, we performed islet grafts. We transplanted islets deficient in either IL-1RI or TNFR1 into wild-type mice and determined the effects on diabetes development.[8,9]

TNFR1 is a member of the so-called death receptor family, and in the right circumstances can signal apoptosis through its intracellular death domain. We grafted islets lacking TNFR1 into NOD4.1 or NOD8.3 mice, and observed blood glucose levels and immune infiltration. In both NOD4.1 and NOD8.3 recipients, TNFR1-deficient islets did not prevent development of hyperglycemia and were destroyed at the same rate as wild-type NOD islets.[8] Histological assessment indicated infiltration of immune cells in both wild-type and TNFR1-deficient grafts. These data indicate that protection from diabetes in TNFR1-deficient NOD mice is not due to prevention of beta cell killing, and rule out a significant role for TNFR1-mediated death signaling in beta cells *in vivo*. The results also indicate that the reduced insulitis in NOD mice lacking TNFR1 is not due to the absence of TNFR1 on beta cells.[8]

Islets lacking IL-1RI were grafted into NOD*scid* mice and their ability to withstand immune attack was tested by adoptive transfer of splenocytes from a diabetic NOD mouse.[9] We observed destruction of islets lacking IL-1RI to the same extent as wild-type islets. These data indicate that there is no significant role of IL-1–dependent killing of beta cells *in vivo*. We also treated some of the recipients of transplanted islets with IL-1R antagonist protein (IL-1Ra) to observe whether systemic blockade of IL-1 could reduce diabetes. While all mice developed diabetes, the islet grafts in mice given IL-1Ra were better preserved than those without IL-1Ra.[9] We conclude that deficiency of IL-1RI in NOD mice does not prevent direct beta cell killing but affects immune system activation.

Regulatory T cells

Type 1 diabetes occurs after failure of immunological tolerance to pancreatic islet self-antigens. Autoreactive T cells are deleted in the thymus by a process known as negative selection. This is an incomplete process, with some autoreactive cells escaping to the periphery. In the periphery, autoreactive cells are controlled by deletion or inactivation and by CD4[+]CD25[+]FoxP3[+] regulatory T cells. It is thought that an imbalance between autoreactive effector T cells and regulatory T cells enhances the likelihood of destruction of pancreatic beta cells and thus type 1 diabetes.

Regulatory T (T_{reg}) cells are a subset of CD4[+] T cells that also express CD25 and the forkhead box protein 3 (FoxP3).[21] T_{reg} cells act by suppressing the proliferation of naive, self-reactive T cells. T_{reg} cells suppress effector T cells through the production of immunosuppressive cytokines and by direct alteration of effector T cells or antigen-presenting cells.[21] FoxP3 deficiency leads to immunodysregulation polyendocrinopathy enteropathy X-linked syndrome (IPEX) in humans and results in development of autoimmune disease in humans and mice.

Regulatory T cells in TNFR1-deficient NOD mice

TNF-α has been implicated in control of T_{reg} cells in autoimmune diseases, including rheumatoid arthritis, Crohn's disease, and type 1 diabetes. The anti-TNF-α antibody increased the number and suppressive function of CD4$^+$CD25$^+$FoxP3$^+$ T cells in patients with rheumatoid arthritis, and similar effects were observed in NOD mice given anti-TNF-α antibody.[22–24] Moreover, a phase II clinical trial of in patients with recent-onset type 1 diabetes showed an improvement in stimulated c-peptide in patients treated with sTNFR (Etanercept).[25] We reasoned that the protection from diabetes observed in NOD mice lacking TNFR1 could be due to an increase in number or function of T_{reg} cells.

We observed an increase in the number and proportion of CD4$^+$CD25$^+$FoxP3$^+$ T_{reg} cells in the absence of TNFR1.[8] To examine the suppressive function of these T_{reg} cells, we determined whether their depletion could abrogate protection from diabetes. NOD8.3 mice develop accelerated diabetes, and NOD8.3 mice lacking TNFR1 did not develop diabetes. When we administered depleting anti-CD4 antibodies to NOD8.3 mice lacking TNFR1, diabetes developed, indicating that the increased numbers of T_{reg} cells in these mice provide protection from diabetes.[8] Together our data indicate that TNF-α has a role in the regulation of CD4$^+$CD25$^+$FoxP3$^+$ T cells, and that in the absence of TNFR1 there is preferential expansion of T_{reg} cells that leads to prevention of diabetes. It is likely that the T_{reg} cells provide an environment that prevents homing of autoreactive T cells to the pancreas. This has also been observed in other organ-specific autoimmune diseases such as experimental autoimmune encephalitis.[26]

In wild-type NOD mice, TNF-α appears at the onset of insulitis, having a suppressive effect on the number and function of T_{reg} cells that results in development of diabetes. In the absence of TNFR1, there is no deleterious effect of TNF-α on T_{reg} cells, resulting in reduced diabetes. We propose that TNF-α signals through TNFR2, which is constitu-

tively expressed at higher levels on T_{reg} cells, leading to their expansion.[8]

Regulatory T cells in IL-RI–deficient mice

IL-1β is produced as a result of activation of the NLRP3 inflammasome. The preclinical prodrome in type 1 diabetes is characterized by a proinflammatory phenotype, including activated NF-κB in dendritic cells and IL-1β overexpression.[27] To a large extent, the effects of IL-1β in development of diabetes have focused on its toxic effects on pancreatic beta cells. However, our data indicate that in NOD mice IL-1β is produced by effector T cells and inhibits the capacity of T_{reg} cells to inhibit effector cells.[28]

We identified a role for IL-1β in the proliferation of CD4$^+$CD25$^+$ T cells, and in the development of CD4$^+$CD25$^+$FoxP3$^+$ T cells. IL-1β inhibited CD4$^+$CD25$^+$ cell-mediated suppression of CD4$^+$CD25$^-$ cells. This resulted in dilution of CD4$^+$CD25$^+$FoxP3$^+$ cells through expansion of CD4$^+$CD25$^+$FoxP3$^-$ effector/memory cells. In NOD mice, higher levels of IL-1β production by splenocytes or macrophages resulted in a reduced proportion of CD25$^+$FoxP3$^+$ cells as mice aged.[28] Therefore IL-1β promotes resistance to suppression by T_{reg} cells, thus reducing the ability of T_{reg} cells to control autoreactivity.[28] This appears to be due to an inability of T_{reg} cells to contain the expression of proinflammatory cytokines, including IL-6, TNF-α, and IL-17, by effector T cells, or by antigen-presenting cells.[28]

The effect of deficiency of IL-1RI on diabetes in NOD mice is minor, indicating that IL-1–mediated suppression of T_{reg} cells is just one of an array of defects in immune regulation. Our results may explain the disappointing results from the two clinical studies of IL-1 inhibition in newly diagnosed type 1 diabetes patients recently reported by Mandrup-Poulsen and Moran (at the 2012 American Diabetes Association meeting). It remains possible that the use of anti-IL-1 antibody to restore the ability of T_{reg} cells to suppress effector cells could be combined with other therapies to reverse type 1 diabetes.[29]

Conclusions

Our results indicate that cytokines such as IL-1 and TNF-α are important in development of diabetes, though not in the way that was originally proposed. We have shown that these cytokines are not required for direct beta cell killing. Instead, we propose that beta cells are primarily destroyed by granule-mediated cytotoxicity as a result of direct contact with CD8$^+$ T cells. Our results show a negative effect of TNF-α and IL-1 on development and function of T_{reg} cells, and indicate that blockade of these cytokines may have beneficial effects on immune regulation in type 1 diabetes.

Acknowledgments

We acknowledge the contribution of Eveline Angstetra, Janette Allison, Sebastien Bertin-Maghit, Dimeng Pang, and Brendan O'Sullivan to the generation of primary data described in this review. This work was supported by a National Health and Medical Research Council of Australia (NHMRC) Program Grant (APP516700), NHMRC Project Grants (APP502605 and APP1034033), and fellowships from the NHMRC (HET) and the Juvenile Diabetes Research Foundation (KLG and BK). This work was supported in part by the Victorian Government's Operational Infrastructure Support Program.

Conflicts of interest

The authors declare no conflicts of interest.

References

1. Barker, J.M. *et al.* 2004. Prediction of autoantibody positivity and progression to type 1 diabetes: Diabetes Autoimmunity Study in the Young (DAISY). *J. Clin. Endocrinol. Metab.* **89:** 3896–3902.
2. Nakayama, M. *et al.* 2005. Prime role for an insulin epitope in the development of type 1 diabetes in NOD mice. *Nature* **435:** 220–223.
3. Krishnamurthy, B. *et al.* 2006. Responses against islet antigens in NOD mice are prevented by tolerance to proinsulin but not IGRP. *J. Clin. Invest.* **116:** 3258–3265.
4. Coppieters, K.T. *et al.* 2012. Demonstration of islet-autoreactive CD8 T cells in insulitic lesions from recent onset and long-term type 1 diabetes patients. *J. Exp. Med.* **209:** 51–60.
5. Rowe, P.A. *et al.* 2011. The pancreas in human type 1 diabetes. *Semin. Immunopathol.* **33:** 29–43.
6. Bertin-Maghit, S. *et al.* 2011. Interleukin-1beta produced in response to islet autoantigen presentation differentiates T-helper 17 cells at the expense of regulatory T-cells: implications for the timing of tolerizing immunotherapy. *Diabetes* **60:** 248–257.
7. Thomas, H.E. *et al.* 2009. Beta cell apoptosis in diabetes. *Apoptosis* **14:** 1389–1404.
8. Chee, J. *et al.* 2011. TNF receptor 1 deficiency increases regulatory T cell function in nonobese diabetic mice. *J. Immunol.* **187:** 1702–1712.
9. Thomas, H.E. *et al.* 2004. IL-1 receptor deficiency slows

10. progression to diabetes in the NOD mouse. *Diabetes* **53:** 113–121.
10. Thomas, H.E. *et al.* 1998. IFN-gamma action on pancreatic beta cells causes class I MHC upregulation but not diabetes. *J. Clin. Invest.* **102:** 1249–1257.
11. Aggarwal, B.B. 2003. Signalling pathways of the TNF superfamily: a double-edged sword. *Nat. Rev. Immunol.* **3:** 745–756.
12. Chen, X. *et al.* 2007. Interaction of TNF with TNF receptor type 2 promotes expansion and function of mouse CD4+CD25+ T regulatory cells. *J. Immunol.* **179:** 154–161.
13. Green, E.A. *et al.* 1998. Local expression of TNF alpha in neonatal NOD mice promotes diabetes by enhancing presentation of islet antigens. *Immunity* **9:** 733–743.
14. Lee, L.F. *et al.* 2005. The role of TNF-alpha in the pathogenesis of type 1 diabetes in the nonobese diabetic mouse: analysis of dendritic cell maturation. *Proc. Natl. Acad. Sci. USA* **102:** 15995–16000.
15. Jacob, C.O. *et al.* 1990. Prevention of diabetes in nonobese diabetic mice by tumor necrosis factor (TNF): similarities between TNF-alpha and interleukin 1. *Proc. Natl. Acad. Sci. USA* **87:** 968–972.
16. Satoh, J. *et al.* 1989. Recombinant human tumor necrosis factor alpha suppresses autoimmune diabetes in nonobese diabetic mice. *J. Clin. Invest.* **84:** 1345–1348.
17. Zhou, R. *et al.* 2010. Thioredoxin-interacting protein links oxidative stress to inflammasome activation. *Nat. Immunol.* **11:** 136–140.
18. Pfleger, C. *et al.* 2008. Association of IL-1ra and adiponectin with C-peptide and remission in patients with type 1 diabetes. *Diabetes* **57:** 929–937.
19. Wang, X. *et al.* 2008. Identification of a molecular signature in human type 1 diabetes mellitus using serum and functional genomics. *J. Immunol.* **180:** 1929–1937.
20. Kagi, D. *et al.* 1999. TNF receptor 1-dependent beta cell toxicity as an effector pathway in autoimmune diabetes. *J. Immunol.* **162:** 4598–4605.
21. Tang, Q. *et al.* 2008. The Foxp3+ regulatory T cell: a jack of all trades, master of regulation. *Nat. Immunol.* **9:** 239–244.
22. Nadkarni, S. *et al.* 2007. Anti-TNF-alpha therapy induces a distinct regulatory T cell population in patients with rheumatoid arthritis via TGF-beta. *J. Exp. Med.* **204:** 33–39.
23. Valencia, X. *et al.* 2006. TNF downmodulates the function of human CD4+CD25hi T-regulatory cells. *Blood* **108:** 253–261.
24. Wu, A.J. *et al.* 2002. Tumor necrosis factor-alpha regulation of CD4+CD25+ T cell levels in NOD mice. *Proc. Natl. Acad. Sci. USA* **99:** 12287–12292.
25. Mastrandrea, L. *et al.* 2009. Etanercept treatment in children with new-onset type 1 diabetes: pilot randomized, placebo-controlled, double-blind study. *Diabetes Care* **32:** 1244–1249.
26. Kohm, A.P. *et al.* 2002. Cutting edge: CD4+CD25+ regulatory T cells suppress antigen-specific autoreactive immune responses and central nervous system

inflammation during active experimental autoimmune encephalomyelitis. *J. Immunol.* **169:** 4712–4716.

27. Poligone, B. *et al.* 2002. Elevated NF-kappaB activation in
nonobese diabetic mouse dendritic cells results in enhanced
APC function. *J. Immunol.* **168:** 188–196.

28. O'Sullivan, B.J. *et al.* 2006. IL-1 beta breaks tolerance

through expansion of CD25+ effector T cells. *J. Immunol.*
176: 7278–7287.

29. Ablamunits, V. *et al.* 2012. Synergistic reversal of type 1 diabetes in NOD mice with anti-CD3 and interleukin-1 blockade: evidence of improved immune regulation. *Diabetes* **61:**
145–154.

Ann. N.Y. Acad. Sci. ISSN 0077-8923

Development of novel genetic cancer vaccines based on membrane-attached β2 microglobulin

Gal Cafri,[1,2] Alon Margalit,[1,3] Esther Tzehoval,[2] Lea Eisenbach,[2] and Gideon Gross[1,3]

[1]Laboratory of Immunology, MIGAL Research Institute, Kiryat Shmona, Israel. [2]Department of Immunology, Weizmann Institute of Science, Rehovot, Israel. [3]Department of Biotechnology, Tel-Hai College, Tel Hai, Israel

Address for correspondence: Gideon Gross, Laboratory of Immunology, MIGAL Research Institute, Kiryat Shmona 11016, Israel. gidi@migal.org.il

Cytotoxic T lymphocytes (CTLs) are the major effector arm of the immune system against tumors. Many tumor-associated antigens (TAAs), known today as potential rejection antigens, were identified by their ability to induce CTL responses. CTLs utilize their clonotypic T cell receptor (TCR) to recognize short antigenic peptides presented on major histocompatibility complex (MHC)-I proteins. These consist of a membrane-attached α heavy chain, which forms the peptide binding pocket, and a noncovalently associated β2m light chain, not anchored to the cell membrane. CTL activation requires that antigenic peptides be presented initially on professional antigen presenting cells (APCs), primarily dendritic cells (DCs). Autologous DCs are a powerful tool for the induction of antitumor responses and are thus widely explored as vehicles for cancer vaccines. Although encouraging evidence for the induction of tumor-specific CTLs by *ex vivo*–manipulated DCs came from numerous animal studies, reproducible objective clinical response in human trials is yet to be demonstrated.

Keywords: β2m; MHC-I; cytotoxic T cells; toll-like receptors; genetic engineering

Presentation of tumor-associated antigen-derived peptides

The density of a given major histocompatibility complex (MHC)–peptide complex on the cell surface determines the degree of T cell responsiveness.[1,2] Cytotoxic T lymphocyte (CTL) priming by a professional antigen presenting cell (APC) generally requires a higher density of specific complexes than that required on the surface of the target cell for activation of an armed effector CTL.[3] Maximal yield of presented peptides derived from encoded proteins is thus a key parameter in the design of cancer vaccines. This rationale has prompted attempts to enhance level of peptide presentation by APCs through genetic manipulations aimed at elevating the actual number of preselected class I–peptide complexes on the cell surface.[4] For example, studies exploring cellular expression of antigenic peptides linked to the N terminus of the class I α chain[5,6] or β2m[7,8] have been reported. When these proteins were expressed on the surface of transfected cells, they were capable of eliciting a specific CTL response following administration of the cells to syngeneic mice. However, broad use of α chain chimeras entails a large collection of expression cassettes, while neither of these two latter designs ensures elevation of complex stability or level on the cell surface, as peptide dissociation from the heavy chain is likely to result in the loss of β2m and consequently of the entire complex.

Membrane-attached β2 microglobulin molecules

In a seminal publication,[9] Yewdell and his colleagues described the intricate process of antigen presentation by MHC-I molecules in quantitative molecular terms. According to this study, proteasomes produce an average of one appropriate MHC-I–peptide precursor out of 40 protein molecules synthesized in the cell ribosomes. Only one out of 50 precursors eventually translocates to the endoplasmic reticulum (ER) to form a stable MHC-I–peptide complex, which exits to the cell surface. These figures amount

doi: 10.1111/nyas.12017

to net efficiency of one MHC-I–peptide complex out of 2000 protein substrates. Protein degradation in the cytosol and peptide trafficking, translocation and final trimming in the ER thus appear bottlenecks, which determine efficacy of MHC-I antigen presentation. Harnessing membrane-attached β_2m as an integral vehicle for delivering chosen, covalently linked antigenic peptides to their class I destination, in an attempt to override these inherent obstacles, bears several obvious advantages on presentation via the conventional MHC-I pathway:

1. Presentation does not depend on proteasomal degradation. In principle, each correctly synthesized polypeptide product inevitably provides its covalently bound peptide as a candidate for presentation.
2. Presentation is TAP independent. Each nascent polypeptide product is immediately targeted to the ER by the β_2m leader peptide.
3. No additional peptide trimming is required. The N-terminus of the peptide is generated through removal of the leader peptide by signal peptidase, whereas the C-terminus is tethered to the linker peptide.
4. Favored complex assembly. Full complex, in fact, comprises two, rather than three components, and its assembly is thus highly favorable

energetically. In addition, membrane attachment of β_2m is expected to increase its availability to heavy chain binding over competing wild-type endogenous β_2m, and is likely to be less dependent on ER chaperons naturally facilitating this step.

5. Increased stability on the cell surface. Peptide dissociation is not followed by peptide and β_2m loss, which later results in heavy chain internalization. Rather, β_2m–peptide polypeptides remain available for heavy chain reassociation through lateral diffusion in the cell membrane. In addition, membrane anchorage may allow recycling of internalized β_2m–peptide, re-forming full complexes in endosomal vesicles.
6. *De novo* complex assembly on the cell surface. Membrane-bound β_2m–peptide is likely to exit to the cell surface independently of class I heavy chains. These free polypeptides would thus constitute a vast membrane pool, capable of pairing with cognate empty heavy chains, including those previously occupied with unrelated peptides.

The first double chimeric β_2m (dcβ_2m) molecules (see Fig. 1) were published six years ago by Margalit *et al.*[10] In these, antigenic peptides were

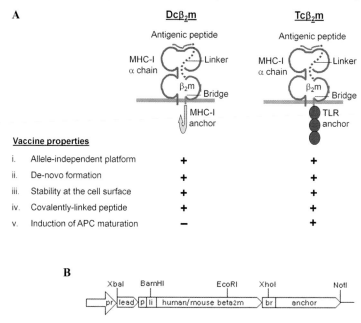

Figure 1. (A) Schemes of the resulting MHC-I molecules at the cell surface, and (B) the basic genetic construct. Abbreviations: pr, promotor; lead, leader peptide; p, antigenic peptide; li, linker; br, bridge. Major restriction sites are indicated.

genetically linked to the N-terminus of β_2m, whereas the C-terminus was genetically anchored to the membrane via a novel peptide bridge followed by the MHC-I transmembrane and cytoplasmic (TC) portions. The dcβ_2m molecules were tested as a platform for cancer vaccines using the B16MO5 (MO5) model. *In vivo*, RMA-S cells transfected with dcβ_2m carrying the MO5 binding peptides OVA$_{257–264}$ or TRP-2$_{181–188}$ elicited stronger CTL response and conferred better tumor protection against MO5 than peptide-saturated parental cells. Furthermore, cells expressing dcβ_2m carrying OVA$_{257–264}$ were significantly superior to OVA$_{257–264}$-carrying cells in their ability to inhibit the growth of pre-established MO5 tumors.

Although dcβ_2m was highly efficient in mediating CTLs induction, it has no known influence on the maturation stage of APCs expressing it. To overcome this shortcoming we designed a second set of chimeric β_2m constructs (Tcβ_2m, see Fig. 1). These were designed to combine optimal presentation of the genetically linked peptide with the stimulation of APC maturation, regulatory T (T$_{reg}$) cell suppression, and Th1-mediated APC conditioning, all mediated by Toll-like receptor (TLR) signaling domains that were incorporated as the β_2m anchor portion. All these effects, in addition to optimal peptide-presentation, were to be imparted in parallel through the product of a single gene. Such a combination has several unique advantages over the first generation molecules:

1. The coupling of a potent and sustained antigenic stimulus with signals required for T$_{reg}$ cell inhibition and for full APC maturation toward CTL priming may suppress possible CTL tolerance to tumor antigens and exert a synergistic effect on the magnitude of the anticipated response.
2. The design entirely precludes the use of adjuvants, which may cause adverse side effects.
3. TLR agonists employed as adjuvants strongly promote APC maturation. However, apart from the associated side effects, it is the persistence of their induced signaling that is necessary for breaking T$_{reg}$-mediated CTL tolerance, and this effect is hard to attain in regular immunization.

In a paper published a year ago,[11] we tested the function of these chimeric molecules in two mouse APC cell lines. We focused on two members of the mouse TLR family, TLR4 and TLR2, that naturally localize to the plasma membrane. We examined different structural and functional aspects of the engraftment of the TIR domain of these TLRs onto the β_2m scaffold. We showed that the encoded peptide–β_2m–TLR polypeptides are expressed at the cell surface, pair with endogenous heavy chains, stabilize MHC-I products, prompt efficient peptide-specific T cell recognition, and confer a constitutively activated phenotype on the transfected cells. Table 1 summarizes our

Table 1. Induction of APC maturation through Tcβ_2m mRNA: list of cell lines and primary cells activated following mRNA transfection

Cells	Origin	mRNA	Induction of cytokine production	Elevation of costimulatory molecules
DC2.4	Mouse Langerhans cell line	caTLR4/2	Yes	Yes
RAW264.7	Mouse macrophage cell line	caTLR4/2	Yes	No
XS52	Mouse dendritic cell line	caTLR4	Yes	Yes
A20	Mouse B cell lymphoma	caTLR4	Yes	ND
THP-I	Human monocytic cell line	caTLR4	Yes	ND
K562	Human myelogenous leukemia	caTLR4	Yes	Yes
Mouse DCs	BM-derived mouse DCs	caTLR4	Yes	Yes
Human DCs	Monocyte-derived human DCs	caTLR4	Yes	Yes

ABBREVIATIONS: CaTLR4/2, Tcβ_2m carrying the TLR4 or TLR2 anchor; BM, bone marrow; DCs, dendritic cells; ND, not determined.

experiments with a panel of mouse and human cell lines and primary cells, showing that the mere transfection of Tcβ$_2$m mRNA, but not irrelevant mRNA, induces cytokine production and upregulates costimulatory molecules. Our results provide evidence that the product of a single recombinant gene can couple MHC peptide presentation to TLR-mediated signaling and offer a safe, economical, and highly versatile modality for a novel category of genetic CTL-inducing vaccines.

Summary

Active vaccination is extensively investigated in the field of cancer immunotherapy. The development of new approaches for improving vaccine efficacy is of main importance for achieving better clinical results. The chimeric β$_2$m platform offers a flexible and modular tool for particularly high MHC-I presentation of tumor-associated peptides coupled to APC activation. Ongoing experiments evaluating the ability of Tcβ$_2$m to confer tumor protection and suppress tumor growth *in vivo* are currently underway.

Conflicts of interest

The authors declare no conflicts of interest.

References

1. Levitsky, V. *et al.* 1996. The life span of major histocompatibility complex-peptide complexes influences the efficiency of presentation and immunogenicity of two class I-restricted cytotoxic T lymphocyte epitopes in the Epstein-Barr virus nuclear antigen 4. *J. Exp. Med.* **183:** 915–926.

2. Tsomides, T.J. *et al.* 1994. Naturally processed viral peptides recognized by cytotoxic T lymphocytes on cells chronically infected by human immunodeficiency virus type 1. *J. Exp. Med.* **180:** 1283–1293.

3. Reis e Sousa, C. 2001. Dendritic cells as sensors of infection. *Immunity* **14:** 495–498.

4. Gross, G. & Margalit, A. 2007. Targeting tumor-associated antigens to the MHC class I presentation pathway. *Endocr. Metab. Immune Disord. Drug Targets* **7:** 99–109.

5. Mottez, E. *et al.* 1995. Cells expressing a major histocompatibility complex class I molecule with a single covalently bound peptide are highly immunogenic. *J. Exp. Med.* **181:** 493–502.

6. Lone, Y.C. *et al.* 1998. In vitro induction of specific cytotoxic T lymphocytes using recombinant single-chain MHC class I/peptide complexes. *J. Immunother.* **21:** 283–294.

7. Uger, R.A. & B.H. Barber. 1998. Creating CTL targets with epitope-linked beta 2-microglobulin constructs. *J. Immunol.* **160:** 1598–1605.

8. Tafuro, S. *et al.* 2001. Reconstitution of antigen presentation in HLA class I-negative cancer cells with peptide-beta2m fusion molecules. *Eur. J. Immunol.* **31:** 440–449.

9. Princiotta, M.F. *et al.* 2003. Quantitating protein synthesis, degradation, and endogenous antigen processing. *Immunity* **18:** 343–354.

10. Margalit, A. *et al.* 2006. Induction of antitumor immunity by CTL epitopes genetically linked to membrane-anchored beta2-microglobulin. *J. Immunol.* **176:** 217–224.

11. Cafri, G. *et al.* 2011. Coupling presentation of MHC class I peptides to constitutive activation of antigen-presenting cells through the product of a single gene. *Int. Immunol.* **23:** 453–461.

Ann. N.Y. Acad. Sci. ISSN 0077-8923

Genomic evaluation of HLA-DR3$^+$ haplotypes associated with type 1 diabetes

Neeraj Kumar,[1] Gurvinder Kaur,[1] Nikhil Tandon,[2] Uma Kanga,[1] and Narinder Mehra[1]

[1]Department of Transplant Immunology and Immunogenetics, [2]Department of Endocrinology and Metabolism, All India Institute of Medical Sciences, New Delhi, India

Address for correspondence: Narinder Mehra, Department of Transplant Immunology and Immunogenetics, All India Institute of Medical Sciences, Ansari Nagar, New Delhi-110029, India. narin98@hotmail.com

We have defined three sets of HLA-DR3$^+$ haplotypes that provide maximum risk of type 1 disease development in Indians: (1) a diverse array of B8-DR3 haplotypes, (2) A33-B58-DR3 haplotype, and (3) A2-B50-DR3 occurring most predominantly in this population. Further analysis has revealed extensive diversity in B8-DR3 haplotypes, particularly at the HLA-A locus, in contrast to the single fixed HLA-A1-B8-DR3 haplotype (generally referred to as AH8.1) reported in Caucasians. However, the classical AH8.1 haplotype was rare and differed from the Caucasian counterpart at multiple loci. In our study, HLA-A26-B8-DR3 (AH8.2) was the most common B8-DR3 haplotype constituting >50% of the total B8-DR3 haplotypes. Further, A2-B8-DR3 contributed the maximum risk (RR = 48.7) of type 1 diabetes, followed by A2-B50-DR3 (RR = 9.4), A33-B58-DR3 (RR = 6.6), A24-B8-DR3 (RR = 4.5), and A26-B8-DR3 (RR = 4.2). Despite several differences, the disease-associated haplotypes in Indian and Caucasian populations share a frozen DR3-DQ2 block, suggesting a common ancestor from which multiple haplotypes evolved independently.

Keywords: HLA; haplotype; type 1 diabetes

Introduction

Type 1 diabetes (T1D) results from the destruction of insulin-producing islet β cells of Langerhans over a prolonged period of time leading to insulin deficiency. Its long-term complications include cardiovascular disease, blindness, and kidney dysfunction. It has been suggested that the inflammatory mediators contribute to the induction and amplification of the immune reaction against the β cells, leading to their destruction, prolonged suppression of function, inhibition of stimulation of β cell regeneration, and peripheral insulin resistance. These different consequences of inflammation occur during different phases of the course of T1D and might be influenced by patients' genetic makeups, leading to disease heterogeneity.[1] Over the last decade, the incidence of T1D has shown a rapid increase, with varying rates among different populations, the highest being in European countries and the lowest in Asian populations.[2] Genetic factors play a major role, as suggested by the reported higher concor-

dance of disease in monozygotic twins (30–50%) than that in dizygotic twins (4.8–27%) and in siblings (4.4–12.5%).[3,4] The major histocompatibility complex (MHC) region in humans is known to harbor genes that contribute more than 50% of the genetic risk toward T1D, mediated primarily by HLA-DR3-DQ2 or DR4-DQ8, or both together. Recently, genome-wide association studies conducted under the Type 1 Diabetes Genetic Consortium (T1DGC), involving a large number of samples representing variable ethnicities, have enabled the discovery of various loci that contribute to T1D susceptibility, including loci within the MHC. HLA genotyping, studies revealed that despite the increasing incidence of disease in the last few decades, the percentage of cases carrying the high-risk HLA genotypes, namely HLA-DR3/DR4-DQB1*03:02, appears to be decreasing, particularly in patients with younger age at disease onset (≤10 years). It has been suggested that disease penetrance might be increasing for both DR3/DR4 and non-DR3/DR4 genotypes, but with a larger proportion of

doi: 10.1111/nyas.12019

non-DR3/DR4 individuals.[5] The T1DGC study also highlights the importance of non-HLA genes and the influence of changing environment on disease development. Currently, over 50 non-HLA regions are reported to significantly influence the risk for type 1 diabetes (http://www.t1dbase.org).

The major histocompatibility complex

The MHC region contains highly polymorphic genes that form separate clusters, referred to in humans as HLA class I (HLA-A, -B, -C) and class II (HLA-DR, -DQ, -DP) regions. The two regions are separated by another cluster of un-related genes, class III, that include complement genes (C4, C2, and Bf), cytokine genes (TNF-α, LTA, LTB), and several other immune-associated genes (MIC-A, MIC-B, heat shock proteins), many of which exert important influence on autoim-mune disease susceptibility. The strongest associ-ations with T1D have been observed with HLA class II determinants HLA-DRB1, DQA1, and DQB1 that account for approximately 40% out of the total ge-netic risk for disease development.[6] Genes in the HLA region display a significant degree of linkage disequilibrium (LD) of alleles at different loci. Ef-forts to establish their individual contribution have not yielded clear-cut information and therefore as-sociation of HLA alleles with the disease must be considered as haplotype specific and not allele spe-cific. In addition to the class II region, genetic vari-ations in HLA class I and class III regions have been reported to modify the disease susceptibil-ity.[7,8] The HLA class I–mediated CD8⁺ T cell re-sponse against islet cell antigens plays a central role in diabetes pathogenesis. It has been reported that β cell toxicity mediated by these cells is governed by the HLA-A2 molecule presenting the insulin B10–B18 peptide.[9] Recently, the HLA-A*24 class I gene has been reported to confer significant risk to disease with an early onset.[10] The study showed that a patient-derived PPI(3–11)-specific CD8⁺ T cell clone acquires a proinflammatory phenotype and is able to kill surrogate β cells as well as hu-man HLA-A*24⁺ islet cells *in vitro*. These results raise the possibility that while class II molecules confer susceptibility to autoimmunity, HLA class I confer-specific susceptibility to type 1 diabetes. It is possible that some unknown genes may also have a critical role in influencing disease suscep-tibility. In European populations, T1D has been shown to be associated mainly with HLA-DR3 or DR4, or both. While in Northern European popu-lations the strongest association is with DR3/DR4 heterozygotes, in Southern Europeans, such as the Basques, the greatest risk to T1D is due to the presence of HLA-DR3 in either a homozygous or heterozygous state.[11] Family-based studies in-dicate that DQA1*05:01-DQB1*02:01 (DQ2) and DQA1*03:01-DQBl*03:02 (DQ8) haplotypes are transmitted to more than 80% of Caucasian di-abetic children, and individuals with the high-est risk for T1D express both of these predispos-ing haplotypes, which are in strong linkage with DRB1*03:01 (DR3) and with DRBl*04:01/02(DR4), respectively.[12,13] Such individuals have been referred to as DR3/DR4 or DQ2/DQ8 heterozygotes. Ap-proximately 40% of diabetic children have been re-ported to carry these genotypes, compared with only ∼2% of healthy children. Accordingly, individuals carrying these high-risk haplotypic combinations have an overall ∼5% absolute risk of developing T1D, which goes up to ∼20% in affected fam-ilies.[14,15] Other HLA haplotypes, for example DRB1*15:01-DQA1*01:02-DQB1*06:02, have con-sistently been reported to confer protection from the disease in almost all populations. Further, the presence of HLA-DRB1*04:03 in an individual has been shown to provide a dominant-protective ef-fect, as it alters the diabetes risk when associated with the high-risk HLA-DQA1*03:01-DQB1*03:02 haplotypes.[16]

The patients included in our study represent the North Indian Hindu population belonging to the North Indian states of Uttar Pradesh, Punjab, Haryana, and Delhi. HLA-DR3 alone was found to provide the greatest risk of developing T1D, with al-most nil or insignificant role of HLA-DR4.[17] One of the reasons for the lack of DR4 association with T1D in the Indian population could be the dominant pro-tective effect conferred by DRB1*04:03 that exists as the predominant DR4 subtype in this population, instead of the positively associated DRB1*04:05 or *04:01 alleles.[18] Table 1 gives a summary of the HLA alleles and haplotypes associated with variable risk in different populations.

Extended MHC haplotypes

The MHC region exhibits strong and extended linkage disequilibrium with occurrence of haplo-types that are conserved for up to 3.2 Mb from

Table 1. T1D-associated HLA class II alleles and haplotypes in various population groups

HLA	Risk	Population
Alleles		
HLA-DRB1*03	High	North Indians and most populations
HLA-DRB1*04	High/low	Caucasians/North Indians
HLA-DRB1*15:01	Protective	North Indians and most populations
DRB1*03/DRB1*04 heterozygote	High	Most populations
DRB1-DQB1 haplotypes		
*03:01–*02:01	High	North Indians and most populations
*04:01–*03:02	High/moderate	Most populations/North Indians
*04:05–*03:02	High/moderate	Most populations/North Indians
*04:04–*03:02	High/moderate	Most populations/North Indians
*09:01–*03:03	Moderate	Chinese, Japanese, Koreans
*07:01–*02:01	Moderate	Blacks
*04:03–*03:02	Protective	North Indians, Caucasians
*11:01–*03:01	Protective	North Indians, Caucasians, Koreans
*15:01–*06:01/02	Protective	North Indians and most populations

HLA-DRB1 to HLA-A locus, as revealed by microsatellite data, complement gene typing, and allelic determination of HLA-DR/DQ, HLA-B, HLA-C, and HLA-A loci.[19] On average, about one-third to half of the Caucasian MHC haplotypes are fixed for about 1 Mb region between HLA-DR/DQ and HLA-B loci. Several studies have suggested that extended or ancestral MHC haplotypes provide an even greater risk to develop autoimmunity compared to individual alleles of any single gene.[20,21] Such extended haplotypes, however, make it difficult to define specific loci that contribute to diabetes risk beyond HLA alleles. Interestingly, the ancestral haplotype AH8.1 (HLA-A1-B8-DR3) is associated not only with T1D, but also with a number of other autoimmune diseases in Caucasians.[22] AH8.1 is extremely conserved up to 9 Mb from HLA-DRB1 to the telomere[23] and occurs with a population frequency of ∼9%, which increases two times in T1D patients.[21] In the French Basque population another DR3 haplotype (A30-B18-Cw5-DR3) has been reported to confer the high diabetes risk.[24] This haplotype is uncommon in most Caucasian populations and thus has a minor contribution to T1D risk. Case-control studies have, however, linked the presence of this haplotype to the development of T1D in children at less than 10 years of age.[25] In the North Indian population, multiple HLA-B8-DR3 haplotypes have

been encountered, all of which are conserved between HLA-B8 and HLA-DR3 but differ remarkably at the HLA-A locus. Of these, A26-B8-DR3, referred to as AH8.2, is the most common haplotype, occurring with a population frequency of 1.48% that increases to 6.2% in patients with T1D (RR = 4.2). Other B8-DR3 haplotypes observed in the North Indian population include A24-B8-DR3, A1-B8-DR3, A11-B8-DR3, A31-B8-DR3, A2-B8-DR3, A3-B8-DR3, A33-B8-DR3, and Ax-B8-DR3. These are shown in Figure 1 with their individual frequencies in patients and the healthy population, along with their relative risk conferred by each of them.

The Caucasian classical HLA-A1-B8-DR3 haplotype is extremely rare in North Indians (frequency ∼0.35%) and shows differences at several loci, including those at HLA-C and DRB3 and central MHC region genes. Similar differences are observed in all of the other B8-DR3 haplotypes observed in our study compared with the Caucasian AH8.1 haplotype. For example, the Indian B8-DR3 haplotypes are characterized by the presence of HLA-Cw*07:02, HLA-DRB3*02:02, HSP70–21267A, TNFA-308G, TNFa 105, C4A-1, and BF*FB, while the Caucasian AH8.1 haplotype is characterized by the presence of HLA-Cw*07:01, HLA-DRB3*01:01, HSP70–21267G, TNFA-308A, TNFa 99, C4A-0, and BF*S. The

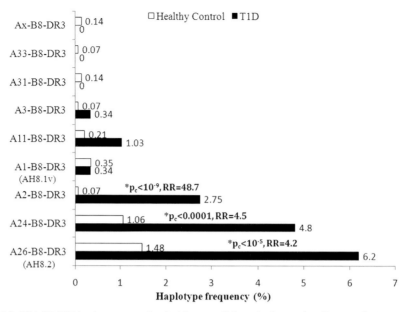

Figure 1. Multiple HLA-B8-DR3 haplotypes associated with type 1 diabetes in the North Indian population.

variant A1-B8-DR3 haplotype has, therefore, been referred to (by us) as AH8.1v and it is not disease associated.

In addition to the multiple B8-DR3 haplotypes, two other haplotypes, namely A2-B50-DR3 (AH50.2; RR = 9.4) and A33-B58-DR3 (AH58.1; RR = 6.6), are associated with T1D in the North Indian population. When we compared the distribution of these haplotypes based on the disease onset, the association of B8-DR3 haplotypes was more prominent in patients with later onset of disease (>10 years). This highlights the role of class I or central MHC genes in disease susceptibility. It is interesting to note that the A33-B58-DR3 haplotype also shows positive disease association in Mongoloid racial groups, including the Chinese.[26] On the other hand, the A2-B50-DR3 haplotype occurs most predominantly in the North Indian population and shows statistically significant association both with T1D[27] as well as Celiac disease.[28] The exact origin of this haplotype is not known, although it has been reported in the Middle East populations and also in some Caucasian groups, albeit with a low frequency (www.allelefrequencies.net). These results support the hypothesis that the Indian population is in the intermediary zone between Caucasoids in the West and Mongoloid in the East and is characterized by alleles and haplotypes of both major groups and harbors various other novel alleles and unique

haplotypes. It is important to note that the Indian population has undergone several waves of human migration from various ethnic groups leading to intense racial admixture and diversification of their genetic architecture.

Evolution/selection of AH8s in North India: a hypothesis

Dominant selection of AH8.2 over AH8.1 in North Indians is analogous to the dominant selection of AH8.1 in Caucasians. In the latter, AH8.1 haplotype has recently been shown to confer protection against progression to bacterial infections as evidenced by the delayed bacterial colonization in cystic fibrosis.[29] This could at least in part explain its high frequency in Caucasian populations. It is conceivable that novel haplotypes generated through multiple recombination events and selection may eventually prove to be beneficial to the population against a recently introduced pathogen. Natural selection favors survival of a population against prevalent infections and/or environmental challenges so that individuals could survive at least up to a reproductive stage, even if it gradually leads to the development of autoimmune disorders at later stages.[30]

Based on the above, our proposal is a hypothetical model of the origin and divergence of B8-DR3+ haplotypes (Fig. 2). It is possible that the two major haplotypes, namely AH8.1 in Caucasians and

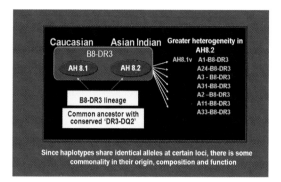

Figure 2. A hypothetical model for the origin and divergence of autoimmunity favoring DR3+ haplotypes in North Indian populations.

AH8.2 in Indians, evolved independently from a common ancestor since they both share HLA-B and DR/DQ alleles, while differing at several other loci. Consequently, the DR3-DQ2 region seems to have remained conserved among these two primordial haplotypes. One explanation could be based on the survival advantage of AH8.2 in Indians as a result of vigorous immune responses to pathogens and/or environmental challenges that might have gradually caused further mutations and selection of the other related haplotypes, including the AH8.1v (variant). Alternatively, Indian populations being more ancestral, environmental stimuli have had ample opportunity to influence diversification of disease-associated B8-DR3 haplotypes. Further, AH8.1 may be a recent entry in the human race and may not have had sufficient time to diversify.

Our hypothesis is consistent with the proposed suggestion that a DNA segment derived from an ancestral haplotype is transferred into a number of diverse and widely distributed haplotypes by recombination, and that certain recombinant haplotypes have subsequently expanded in frequency across populations.[31] Interestingly, it seems that one of these ancient recombinations occurred within the TNF-cluster, as evidenced by the fact that the TNF2 and LTA 252G alleles display a strong linkage disequilibrium in Caucasian populations,[32] which was not observed in North Indians. All of the Indian DR3-B8 haplotypes had the wild-type TNF1 allele, besides the LTA 252G. These observations support the suggestion that ancestral DR3-DQ2 "blocks" have been shuffled into different MHC haplotypes. The expansion of the resultant novel haplotypes might relate to selection for resistance to disease

by offering an evolutionary advantage for HLA class II functions and peptide-binding specificities. The spread of the DR3-DQ2 ancestral segment by inter-haplotype exchange may also have been driven by selection. Whether the maintenance of polymorphic conserved and common blocks such as the DR-DQ segment is due to suppression of recombination, or selection, is not clear. Existence of such a selection pressure on the Indian DR3 haplotypes is also illustrated by their unique combination of HLA-DRB1-DRB3 alleles, compared with other populations. The Caucasian AH8.1 always has the DRB1*03:01–DRB3*01:01 haplotype, while all Indian DR3+ haplotypes have DRB1*03:01–DRB3*02:02. In Black populations, the DR3+ haplotypes are characterized by DRB1*03:02–DRB3*02:02. It has been reported that ancient, highly divergent MHC haplotypes appear to be evolving independently, except for a specific sequence in the peptide-binding groove and rare block shuffling.[33] However, more detailed anthropological studies based on multi-SNP analyses are needed to answer why, where, and how these different haplotypes arose, as well as what the functional implications are of the independent evolution of various disease-associated haplotypes.

Acknowledgments

The authors wish to thank the Department of Biotechnology (DBT), Ministry of Science and Technology, Government of India, and the Indian Council of Medical Research (ICMR) for providing financial support for the study.

Conflicts of interest

The authors declare no conflicts of interest.

References

1. Eizirik, D.L. *et al.* 2009. The role of inflammation in insulitis and β-cell loss in type 1 diabetes. *Nat. Rev. Endocrinol.* **5:** 219–226.
2. Karvonen, M. *et al.* 2000. Incidence of childhood type 1 diabetes worldwide. Diabetes Mondiale (DiaMond) Project Group. *Diabetes Care* **23:** 1516–1526.
3. Davis, J.A. 1996. Insulin dependent diabetes mellitus in twins. Differences between monozygotic and dizygotic twins may need to be taken into account. **312:** 313–314.
4. European Consortium for IDDM Genome Studies. 2001. A Genomewide scan for type 1–diabetes susceptibility in Scandinavian families: identification of new loci with evidence of interactions. *AJHG* **69:** 1301–1313.

5. Steck, A.K. *et al.* 2011. Stepwise or linear decrease in penetrance of type 1 diabetes with lower-risk HLA genotypes over the past 40 years. *Diabetes* **60:** 1045–1049.

6. Jones, E.Y. *et al.* 2006. MHC class II proteins and disease: a structural perspective. *Nat. Rev. Immunol.* **6:** 271–282.

7. Nejentsev, S. *et al.* 2007. Localization of type 1 diabetes susceptibility to the MHC class I genes HLA-B and HLA-A. *Nature* **450:** 887–892.

8. Skanes, V.M. *et al.* 1986. Class III alleles and high-risk MHC haplotypes in type I diabetes mellitus, Graves' disease and Hashimoto's thyroiditis. *Mol. Biol. Med.* **3:** 143–157.

9. Pinkse, G.G. *et al.* 2006. Independent and reproducible identification of proinsulin epitopes of CD8 T cells- report of the IDS T cell workshop committee. *Ann. N.Y. Acad. Sci.* **1079:** 19–23.

10. Kronenberg, D. *et al.* 2012. Circulating preproinsulin signal peptide-specific CD8 T cells restricted by the susceptibility molecule HLA-A24 are expanded at onset of type 1 diabetes and kill β-cells. *Diabetes* **61:** 1752–1759.

11. Bilbao, J.R. *et al.* 2006. Conserved extended haplotypes discriminate HLA-DR3-homozygous Basque patients with type 1 diabetes mellitus and celiac disease. *Genes Immun.* **7:** 550–554.

12. Cerna, M. *et al.* 2003. HLA in Czech adult patients with autoimmune diabetes mellitus: comparison with Czech children with type 1 diabetes and patients with type 2 diabetes. *Eur. J. Immunogenet.* **30:** 401–407.

13. Buc, M. *et al.* 2006. Associations between HLA class II alleles and type 1 diabetes mellitus in the Slovak population. *Endocr. Regul.* **40:** 1–6.

14. Chowdhury, T.A. *et al.* 1999. The aetiology of type I diabetes. *Clin. Baillieres. Best. Pract. Res. Clin. Endocrinol. Metabol.* **13:** 181–195.

15. Concannon, P. *et al.* 2005. Type 1 diabetes: evidence for susceptibility loci from four genome-wide linkage scans in 1,435 multiplex families. *Diabetes* **54:** 2995–3001.

16. Van der Auwera, B. *et al.* 1995. DRB1*0403 protects against IDDM in Caucasians with the high-risk heterozygous DQA1*0301-DQB1*0302/DQA1*0501-DQB1*0201 genotype. Belgian Diabetes Registry. *Diabetes* **44:** 527–530.

17. Mehra, N.K. *et al.* 2007. Biomarkers of susceptibility to type 1 diabetes with special reference to the Indian population. *Indian J. Med. Res.* **125:** 321–344.

18. Jaini, R. *et al.* 2002. Heterogeneity of HLA-DRB1*04 and its associated haplotypes in the North Indian population. *Hum. Immunol.* **63:** 24–29.

19. Cattley, S.K. *et al.* 2000. Further characterization of MHC haplotypes demonstrates conservation telomeric of HLA-A: update of the 4AOH and 10IHW cell panels. *Eur. J. Immunogenet.* **27:** 397–426.

20. Degli-Esposti, M.A. *et al.* 1992. Ancestral haplotypes carry haplotypic and haplospecific polymorphisms of BAT1: possible relevance to autoimmune disease. *Eur. J. Immunogenet.* **19:** 121–126.

21. Alper, C.A. *et al.* 2006. The haplotype structure of the human major histocompatibility complex. *Hum. Immunol.* **67:** 73–84.

22. Price, P. *et al.* 1999. The genetic basis for the association of the 8.1 ancestral haplotype (A1, B8, DR3) with multiple immunopathological diseases. *Immunol. Rev.* **167:** 257–274.

23. Aly, T.A. *et al.* 2008. Analysis of SNPs identifies major type 1A diabetes locus telomeric of the MHC. *Diabetes* **57:** 770–776.

24. Cambon-de Mouzon, A. *et al.* 1982. HLA-A, B, C, DR antigens, Bf, C4 and glyoxalase I (GLO) polymorphisms in French Basques with insulin-dependent diabetes mellitus (IDDM). *Tissue Antigens.* **19:** 366–379.

25. Tait B.D. *et al.* 1995. HLA antigens and age at diagnosis of insulin-dependent diabetes mellitus. *Hum. Immunol.* **42:** 116–122.

26. Feng, M.L. *et al.* 2003. Study on HLA haplotypes in Jiangsu–Zhejiang–Shanghai Han population. *Yi. Chuan. Xue. Bao.* **30:** 584–588.

27. Kanga, U. *et al.* 2004. HLA haplotypes associated with type 1 diabetes mellitus in North Indian children. *Hum. Immunol.* **65:** 47–53.

28. Kaur, G. *et al.* 2002. Pediatric celiac disease in India is associated with multiple DR3-DQ2 haplotypes. *Hum. Immunol.* **63:** 677–682.

29. Aladzsity, I. *et al.* 2011. Analysis of the 8.1 ancestral MHC haplotype in severe, pneumonia-related sepsis. *Clin. Immunol.* **139:** 282–289.

30. Westendorp, R.G.J. 2004. Are we becoming less disposable? *EMBO reports* **5:** 2–6.

31. Prugnolle, F. *et al.* 2005. Pathogen-driven selection and worldwide HLA class I diversity. *Curr. Biol.* **15:** 1022–1027.

32. Gaudieri, S. *et al.* 1997. The major histocompatability complex (MHC) contains conserved polymorphic genomic sequences that are shuffled by recombination to form ethnic-specific haplotypes. *J. Mol. Evol.* **45:** 17–23.

33. Traherne, J.A. *et al.* 2006. Genetic analysis of completely sequenced disease-associated MHC haplotypes identifies shuffling of segments in recent human history. *PLOS Genet.* **2:** e9.

Ann. N.Y. Acad. Sci. ISSN 0077-8923

ANNALS OF THE NEW YORK ACADEMY OF SCIENCES

Issue: *Translational Immunology in Asia-Oceania*

PPE2 protein of *Mycobacterium tuberculosis* may inhibit nitric oxide in activated macrophages

Khalid Hussain Bhat,[1] Arghya Das,[1] Aparna Srikantam,[2] and Sangita Mukhopadhyay[1]

[1]Centre for DNA Fingerprinting and Diagnostics, Nampally, [2]Blue Peter Research Centre (LEPRA Society), Hyderabad, Andhra Pradesh, India

Address for correspondence: Sangita Mukhopadhyay, Laboratory of Molecular Cell Biology, Centre for DNA Fingerprinting and Diagnostics (CDFD), Gruhakalpa Building, Nampally, Hyderabad, Andhra Pradesh 500001, India. sangita@cdfd.org.in

Although the pathophysiological role of PE/PPE proteins of *Mycobacterium tuberculosis* is yet to be fully understood, recent evidence shows that these proteins play important roles in antigenic diversity, as well as in host–pathogen interactions and mycobacterial pathogenesis. Most of the PE/PPE proteins are highly expressed in pathogenic bacteria, pointing to their role in the pathogenesis of mycobacteria. Here, we provide an overview of our work in progress on a specific PPE protein, PPE2 (Rv0256c), which may inhibit nitric oxide (NO) production in activated macrophages. As NO and its by-products are considered to be toxic to bacilli, it is possible that the bacilli recruit Rv0256c in order to inhibit higher production of NO during infection.

Keywords: *M. tuberculosis*; PPE2 protein; nitric oxide; macrophage

Introduction

Tuberculosis (TB) is a global health problem; billions of people are infected and millions die every year.[1] The causative organism of TB *Mycobacterium tuberculosis* has plagued humankind since prehistoric times.[2] *M. tuberculosis* enters the human airways via aerosol droplets from infected patients and is ultimately taken up by lung alveolar macrophages. Macrophages function as antimycobacterial warriors and play crucial roles in regulating host defense responses to kill the invading bacilli.[3] However, the bacilli have evolved a plethora of strategies to bypass and overcome the defense strategies of macrophages to ensure their ability to survive and propagate inside hosts.[4,5] One of the well-known strategies adopted by bacilli is the inhibition of phagosome–lysosome fusion that results in inhibition of acidification of the maturing phagosome, thereby limiting its exposure to degradative enzymes of lysosomes.[6] Other than lysosome-mediated killing, host macrophages induce oxidative burst and produce toxic products such as reactive oxygen species during infection.[7]

Bacilli have also evolved various strategies to reduce the deleterious effects of various free radicals.[4] For example, *ahpC* and *katG* genes overexpressed in mycobacteria during oxidative stress conditions code for catalase-peroxidase and alkyl hydroperoxide reductase (peroxiredoxin) enzymes, respectively, and help to neutralize the free radicals generated by host macrophages.[8] Nitric oxide (NO), generated by inducible NO synthase (iNOS), is also a potent mycobactericidal molecule and, in combination with other reactive oxygen species, produces nitrous oxide (ONOO), which is toxic to intracellular mycobacteria.[9,10] Interestingly, iNOS knock-out mice were found to be more susceptible to mycobacterial infection compared to wild-type mice.[11] Thus, inhibition of NO production could be one of the key virulence steps of mycobacteria to maintain chronic infection in the host.

The proline–glutamic acid (PE) and proline–proline–glutamic acid (PPE) family of proteins became a greater focus of attention when the *M. tuberculosis* genome was first sequenced in 1998.[12] It was observed that almost 10% of the coding capacity of *M. tuberculosis* codes proteins having conserved domains at their N-terminal regions. PE and PPE

doi: 10.1111/nyas.12070

were so named becaused of the presence of multiple repeats at their N-terminal regions.[12] The PE/PPE family is further subdivided based on the sequence similarities among different members.[13] Although the pathophysiological role of PE/PPE proteins of *M. tuberculosis* is yet to be fully understood, recent evidence indicates that these proteins play important roles in antigenic diversity, host–pathogen interactions, and pathogenesis.[14–19]

In this short overview, we provide an overview of our work in progress on PPE2 (Rv0256c), providing preliminary data that are consistent with the possibility that PPE2 inhibits NO production in activated macrophages.

PPE2 effects on NO production

The PPE2 protein was reported to be overexpressed during both NO stress conditions and infection with *M. tuberculosis*, indicating that the protein may play a role in neutralizing NO stress.[20, 21] The expression of the protein in pathogenic bacteria varies in different clinical isolates and therefore might have an important function in the pathogenicity of mycobacteria.[22, 23] Since the protein is upregulated during NO stress and NO plays a crucial role in killing mycobacteria, we have hypothesized that PPE2 might inhibit NO production in macrophages. To study the effect of PPE2 manipulations on macrophage innate responses, in a preliminary experiment we infected RAW 264.7 macrophages with wild-type (WT) or PPE2 knock-out (KO) *M. tuberculosis* CDC1551 strains; the Rv0256c KO is a gene disruption transposon mutant (2163, MT0269, NR-15106, POI: 638) developed by Lamichhane *et al.*[24] In brief, the macrophages are infected with the WT or KO strains at 1:10 multiplicities of infection (MOI) after which production of NO, as well as various cytokines, including IL-10, IL-12, and TNF-α, known to be induced in activated macrophages, are measured 48 h postinfection using a Griess assay (for measurement of NO) and an enzyme immunoassay (for measurement of cytokines).[25] Our initial studies indicate that, although no significant effects on IL-10, IL-12, and TNF-α production are detected, NO production is downregulated in RAW 264.7 macrophages infected with WT but not the KO *M. tuberculosis* strain (Fig. 1, work in progress). These data are consistent with the possibility that PPE2 inhibits NO production in macrophages.

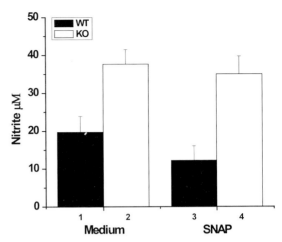

Figure 1. Macrophages infected with the PPE2 (Rv0256c) knock-out (KO) CDC1551 *M. tuberculosis* strain produce more NO compared to wild-type (WT). RAW 264.7 macrophages are infected *in vitro* with WT or KO grown in the absence or presence of SNAP at 1:10 MOI. Levels of nitrite in culture supernatants are measured after 48 h of infection by Griess assay. This figure represents work in progress.

Since earlier microarray studies indicated overexpression of PPE2 during NO stress,[20, 21] we predict that NO production would be inhibited more strongly in macrophages infected with *M. tuberculosis* strains that were preexposed to NO stress. To test this, we are performing experiments in which WT and KO *M. tuberculosis* bacterial cells are grown in the presence of *S*-nitroso-*N*-acetyl-DL-penicillamine (SNAP), a donor of NO that spontaneously releases NO in cultures.[26, 27] The WT and KO bacteria with or without (control) exposure to SNAP are next used to infect RAW 264.7 macrophages. Consistent with our prediction, our results thus far show that SNAP/NO treatment increases PPE2 expression in the WT *M. tuberculosis* bacteria (results not shown). Interestingly, NO production is inhibited to a greater extent (data not shown) in macrophages infected with the WT *M. tuberculosis* exposed to SNAP/NO stress compared with those infected with the control WT *M. tuberculosis*, while no difference in NO production is found between macrophages infected with the KO *M. tuberculosis*, regardless of SNAP exposure (see Fig. 1). These results suggest increased expression of PPE2 during NO stress and possible involvement of PPE2 in inhibition of NO production in macrophages.

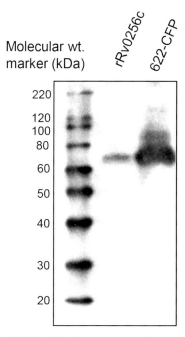

Figure 2. PPE2 (Rv0256c) is secreted in culture supernatant. Clinical *M. tuberculosis* strain is cultured in Sauton's medium supplemented with 0.05% Tween-80. The culture supernatant is concentrated (400 times), resolved on a SDS-PAGE gel, and immunoblotted using a commercially generated anti-PPE2 antibody and HRP-conjugated antirabbit secondary antibody. rRv0256c, recombinant Rv0256c protein; 622-CFP, culture filtrate protein of strain 622. This figure represents work in progress.

PPE2: a secretory protein

To determine the localization of PPE2 in *M. tuberculosis*, we are performing experiments in which PPE2 is overexpressed in the nonpathogenic strain *M. smegmatis*, which does not naturally contain the PPE2 protein. When these cells are fractionated, the protein can be found to be in the soluble, but not cell wall–rich fraction, suggesting that the protein is not localized in the cell wall region. Many PPE proteins are found to be secreted by mycobacteria via the ESX pathway.[17,19,28–30] We therefore hypothesize that the PPE2 protein might also be secreted by *M. tuberculosis*. Initial and ongoing analyses indeed show the presence of PPE2 in culture supernatants of clinical strains of *M. tuberculosis* (Fig. 2, work in progress). Thus, we hypothesize that the protein is present in the cytoplasm of macrophages, owing to the porous nature of phagosome during *M. tuberculosis* infection; it has been observed, for example, that *M. tuberculosis*–containing phagosomes are permeable

to protein up to 70 kDa in size.[31] Thus, the PPE2 protein, 58 kDa in size, is small enough to cross the phagosomal membrane and reach the cytoplasm of the host macrophage where it could ultimately interfere with macrophage signaling cascades involved in iNOS/NO regulation. It is also possible that *M. tuberculosis* can escape from its vacuole to the cytoplasm of infected cells, as shown by van der Wel *et al.*,[32] thus allowing bacilli to secrete the Rv0256c protein directly into the cytoplasm.

In other preliminary studies, we have examined the production of lipopolysaccharide (LPS)-induced NO, as well as of various innate cytokines, following cytoplasmic overexpression of PPE2 in RAW 264.7 macrophages by lipofectamine-mediated transfection (transfection simulates the conditions under which PPE2 is likely secreted by bacilli into the cytoplasm of infected cells). Thus far we have found that the cytoplasmic overexpression of PPE2 in macrophages results in downregulation of LPS-induced NO production, without significantly affecting production of IL-10, IL-12, and TNF-α, compared with macrophages harboring the backbone plasmid alone (data not shown). Although this work is preliminary and ongoing, the experiments carried out so far indicate that PPE2 of *M. tuberculosis* likely plays an important role in inhibition of NO production in activated macrophages. Further investigation is required to understand how *M. tuberculosis* targets PPE2 to inhibit NO production in macrophages.

Summary

The PE/PPE gene family, with 176 open reading frames, is unique to mycobacteria. These proteins are mostly nonessential for growth in culture conditions and are differentially expressed in *M. tuberculosis* during infection. Thus, they are thought to be involved in host–pathogen interaction and pathogenesis of *M. tuberculosis*. We describe here that PPE2 protein expression increases during NO stress and may be involved in downregulation of NO production in activated macrophages. These preliminary findings are being confirmed by experiments *in vitro* with infection of macrophages by PPE2 knock-out *M. tuberculosis* CDC1551 and WT strains and then evaluating and comparing any effects on NO production. If confirmed by additional experiments, possible mechanisms by which the PPE2 protein inhibits NO

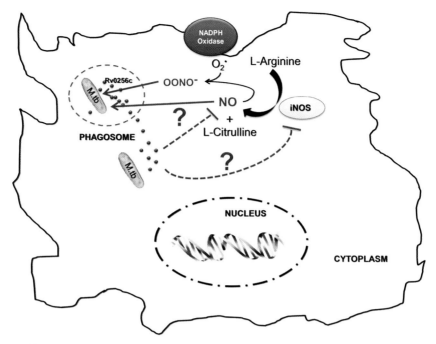

Figure 3. A possible mechanism of action of PPE2 (Rv0256c). NO, a product of iNOS, in combination with ONOO$^-$, is known to be cytotoxic to *M. tuberculosis* and is present inside phagosomes or the cytoplasm of macrophages. Rv0256c secreted by *M. tuberculosis* under NO stress probably resides in the cytoplasm and inhibits NO/iNOS via mechanisms yet to be identified.

synthesis would require further experiments. Preliminary studies to date indicate that inhibition of NO production by Rv0256c may be at the level of iNOS transcription. Since iNOS/NO plays an important role in antimycobacterial immunity, we hope that study of possible mechanisms by which PPE2 inhibits NO production in macrophages (Fig. 3) could ultimately lead to development of new interventional strategies to prevent active tuberculosis disease.

Acknowledgments

We acknowledge the gift of mutant (NR-15106, MT0269) and WT strains (CDC1551) *of M. tuberculosis* from Colorado State University as part of the NIH, NIAID Contract No. HHSN266200400091C, entitled "Tuberculosis Vaccine Testing and Research Materials," awarded to Colorado State University. We are grateful to Prof. V.S. Chauhan (ICGEB, India), and Dr. Pawan Sharma (ICGEB, India), for their kind help and support in carrying out *in vitro* infection experiments at the DBT-funded National Facility for Tuberculosis Research at ICGEB, New Delhi. We thank the Council of Scientific and Industrial Research (CSIR) for the fellowships provided to KHB and AD. This work was supported by a core grant to CDFD from DBT, India.

Conflicts of interest

Part of this work has been applied for patent, S. Mukhopadhyay *et al.* (filed in USA, [USPTO, 31 Aug 2009]).

References

1. Dye, C. *et al.* 1999. Consensus statement. Global burden of tuberculosis: estimated incidence, prevalence, and mortality by country. WHO Global Surveillance and Monitoring Project. *JAMA* **282:** 677–686.
2. Fatkenheuer, G. *et al.* 1999. The return of tuberculosis. *Diagn. Microbiol. Infect. Dis.* **34:** 139–146.
3. Ernst, J. D. 1998. Macrophage receptors for *Mycobacterium tuberculosis. Infect. Immun.* **66:** 1277–1281.
4. Flynn, J. L. & J. Chan. 2003. Immune evasion by *Mycobacterium tuberculosis*: living with the enemy. *Curr. Opin. Immunol.* **15:** 450–455.
5. Gupta, A. *et al.* 2012. Mycobacterium tuberculosis: immune evasion, latency and reactivation. *Immunobiology* **217:** 363–374.
6. Vergne, I. *et al.* 2004. Cell biology of *Mycobacterium tuberculosis* phagosome. *Annu. Rev. Cell. Dev. Biol.* **20:** 367–394.
7. Flynn, J. L. & J. Chan. 2001. Immunology of tuberculosis. *Annu. Rev. Immunol.* **19:** 93–129.

8. Manca, C. *et al.* 1999. Mycobacterium tuberculosis catalase and peroxidase activities and resistance to oxidative killing in human monocytes in vitro. *Infect. Immun.* **67:** 74–79.

9. Chan, J. *et al.* 1992. Killing of virulent *Mycobacterium tuberculosis* by reactive nitrogen intermediates produced by activated murine macrophages. *J. Exp. Med.* **175:** 1111–1122.

10. MacMicking, J., Q. W. Xie & C. Nathan. 1997. Nitric oxide and macrophage function. *Annu. Rev. Immunol.* **15:** 323–350.

11. MacMicking, J. D. *et al.* 1997. Identification of nitric oxide synthase as a protective locus against tuberculosis. *Proc. Natl. Acad. Sci. USA* **94:** 5243–5248.

12. Cole, S. T. *et al.* 1998. Deciphering the biology of *Mycobacterium tuberculosis* from the complete genome sequence. *Nature* **393:** 537–544.

13. Gey van Pittius, N. C. *et al.* 2006. Evolution and expansion of the *Mycobacterium tuberculosis* PE and PPE multigene families and their association with the duplication of the ESAT-6 (esx) gene cluster regions. *BMC Evol. Biol.* **6:** 95.

14. Brennan, M. J. & G. Delogu. 2002. The PE multigene family: a 'molecular mantra' for mycobacteria. *Trends Microbiol.* **10:** 246–249.

15. Tian, C. & X. Jian-Ping. 2010. Roles of PE_PGRS family in *Mycobacterium tuberculosis* pathogenesis and novel measures against tuberculosis. *Microb. Pathog.* **49:** 311–314.

16. Nair, S., A. D. Pandey & S. Mukhopadhyay. 2011. The PPE18 protein of *Mycobacterium tuberculosis* inhibits NF-κB/rel-mediated proinflammatory cytokine production by upregulating and phosphorylating suppressor of cytokine signaling 3 protein. *J. Immunol.* **186:** 5413–5424.

17. Nair, S. *et al.* 2009. The PPE18 of *Mycobacterium tuberculosis* interacts with TLR2 and activates IL-10 induction in macrophage. *J. Immunol.* **183:** 6269–6281.

18. Basu, S. *et al.* 2007. Execution of macrophage apoptosis by PE_PGRS33 of *Mycobacterium tuberculosis* is mediated by Toll-like receptor 2-dependent release of tumor necrosis factor-α. *J. Biol. Chem.* **282:** 1039–1050.

19. Bhat, K. H. *et al.* 2012. Proline-proline-glutamic acid (PPE) protein Rv1168c of *Mycobacterium tuberculosis* augments transcription from HIV-1 long terminal repeat promoter. *J. Biol. Chem.* **287:** 16930–16946.

20. Voskuil, M. I. *et al.* 2003. Inhibition of respiration by nitric oxide induces a *Mycobacterium tuberculosis* dormancy program. *J. Exp. Med.* **198:** 705–713.

21. Honaker, R. W. *et al.* 2009. Unique roles of DosT and DosS in DosR regulon induction and *Mycobacterium tuberculosis* dormancy. *Infect. Immun.* **77:** 3258–3263.

22. Gao, Q. *et al.* 2005. Gene expression diversity among *Mycobacterium tuberculosis* clinical isolates. *Microbiology* **151:** 5–14.

23. Homolka, S. *et al.* 2010. Functional genetic diversity among *Mycobacterium tuberculosis* complex clinical isolates: delineation of conserved core and lineage-specific transcriptomes during intracellular survival. *PLoS Pathog.* **6:** e1000988.

24. Lamichhane, G. *et al.* 2003. A postgenomic method for predicting essential genes at subsaturation levels of mutagenesis: application to *Mycobacterium tuberculosis*. *Proc. Natl. Acad. Sci. USA* **100:** 7213–7218.

25. Mukhopadhyay, S. *et al.* 2002. Macrophage effector functions controlled by Bruton's tyrosine kinase are more crucial than the cytokine balance of T cell responses for microfilarial clearance. *J. Immunol.* **168:** 2914–2921.

26. Lander, H. M. *et al.* 1993. Activation of human peripheral blood mononuclear cells by nitric oxide-generating compounds. *J. Immunol.* **150:** 1509–1516.

27. Field, L. *et al.* 1978. An unusually stable thionitrite from *N*-acetyl-D, L-penicillamine; X-ray crystal and molecular structure of 2-(acetylamino)-2-carboxy-1, 1-dimethylethyl thionitrite. *J. Chem. Soc., Chem. Commun.* 249–250.

28. Abdallah, A. M. *et al.* 2009. PPE and PE_PGRS proteins of *Mycobacterium marinum* are transported via the type VII secretion system ESX-5. *Mol. Microbiol.* **73:** 329–340.

29. Bottai, D. & R. Brosch. 2009. Mycobacterial PE, PPE and ESX clusters: novel insights into the secretion of these most unusual protein families. *Mol. Microbiol.* **73:** 325–328.

30. Sayes, F. *et al.* 2012. Strong immunogenicity and cross-reactivity of *Mycobacterium tuberculosis* ESX-5 type VII secretion -encoded PE-PPE proteins predicts vaccine potential. *Cell Host Microbe.* **11:** 352–363.

31. Teitelbaum, R. *et al.* 1999. Mycobacterial infection of macrophages results in membrane-permeable phagosomes. *Proc. Natl. Acad. Sci. USA* **96:** 15190–15195.

32. van der Wel, N. *et al.* (2007). *M. tuberculosis* and *M. leprae* translocate from the phagolysosome to the cytosol in myeloid cells. *Cell* **129:** 1287–1298.

Ann. N.Y. Acad. Sci. ISSN 0077-8923

ANNALS OF THE NEW YORK ACADEMY OF SCIENCES
Issue: *Translational Immunology in Asia-Oceania*

Corrigendum for Ann. N.Y. Acad. Sci. 2012. 1274: 86–91

Evoli, A., P.E. Alboini, A. Bisonni, A. Mastrorosa & E. Bartocccioni. 2012. Management challenges in muscle-specific tyrosine kinase myasthenia gravis. *Ann. N.Y. Acad. Sci.* 1274: 86–91.

The last author's name in the above-cited article should be spelled Bartoccioni.

doi: 10.1111/nyas.12132

Ann. N.Y. Acad. Sci. ISSN 0077-8923

ANNALS OF THE NEW YORK ACADEMY OF SCIENCES
Issue: *Translational Immunology in Asia-Oceania*

Erratum for Ann. N.Y. Acad. Sci. 2012. 1275: 54–62

Engel, A.G., X-M. Shen, D. Selcen & S. Sine. 2012. New horizons for congenital myasthenic syndromes. *Ann. N.Y. Acad. Sci.* 1275: 54–62.

On page 61 of the above-mentioned article, the paragraph beginning with "Parameters of neuromuscular transmission . . ." just above the heading "CMS caused by defects in DPAGT1" should have been deleted.

The editorial staff of *Annals of the New York Academy of Sciences* regrets this error.

doi: 10.1111/nyas.12133